Facial Skin Disorders

SERIES IN DERMATOLOGICAL TREATMENT

Published in association with the *Journal of Dermatological Treatment*

Already available

Robert Baran, Roderick Hay, Eckart Haneke, Antonella Tosti, *Onychomycosis,* second edition
ISBN 0415385792

Forthcoming

Sakari Reitamo, Thomas A Luger, *Textbook of Atopic Dermatitis*
ISBN 184184246X

Of related interest

Steven R Feldman, Kathy C Phelps, Kelly C Verzino, *Handbook of Dermatologic Drug Therapy*
ISBN 1842142607

Lionel Fry, *Atlas of Dermatology,* fifth edition
ISBN 1842142372

Arthur Jackson, Graham Colver, Rodney PR Dawber, *Cutaneous Cryosurgery,* third edition
ISBN 1841845523

Antonella Tosti, Bianca Maria Piraccini, *Diagnosis and Treatment of Hair Disorders*
ISBN 1841843407

Michael D Zanolli, Steven R Feldman, *Phototherapy Treatment Protocols for Psoriasis and Other Phototherapy-Responsive Dermatoses*, second edition
ISBN 1842142526

Facial Skin Disorders

Ronald Marks FRCP FRCPATH

Emeritus Professor

University of Wales

Cardiff

UK

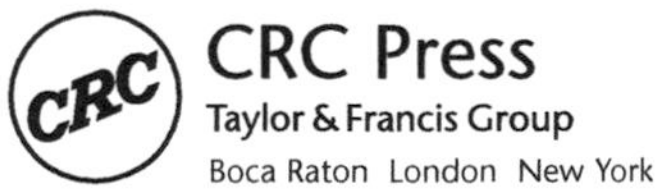

CRC Press
Taylor & Francis Group
Boca Raton London New York

CRC Press is an imprint of the
Taylor & Francis Group, an **informa** business

CRC Press
Taylor & Francis Group
6000 Broken Sound Parkway NW, Suite 300
Boca Raton, FL 33487-2742

First issued in paperback 2019

ISBN-13: 978-1-84184-210-3 (hbk)
ISBN-13: 978-0-367-38939-0 (pbk)

A CIP record for this book is available from the British Library.

Library of Congress Cataloging-in-Publication Data available on application

Visit the Taylor & Francis Web site at
http://www.taylorandfrancis.com

and the CRC Press Web site at
http://www.crcpress.com

Contents

Foreword

Dr Ronald Marks has been intrigued and fascinated for much of his distinguished career by disorders of the face. He has published a multitude of articles and a small library of books on disorders which disfigure the face.

His bona fides for writing this magnum opus reflect his extraordinary talents and capabilities as a teacher, clinician, investigator, publicist, and organizer of international symposia dedicated to the varied and diverse aspects of these common and troubling diseases, including acne, rosacea, seborrheic dermatitis, photoaging, tumors, infections, etc. The uniqueness of this volume as the most comprehensive and complete work on this subject can be attributed, in addition to his vast clinical experience, to his extensive knowledge of the immunologic, molecular, biochemical, histologic, photobiologic, and not least, his psychologic understanding of these common distressing disorders.

This up-to-date text, with its carefully selected, voluminous but relevant references, is directed to a wide readership and is required reading for researchers, clinicians, cosmetic surgeons, and especially educators in academic centers who have a focus on the many and diverse signs and symptoms of facial affliction.

Marks makes the keen and sad observation that funding for these common problems, such as acne and rosacea, has been egregiously feeble, which is certainly the case in the USA where it will come as a shock that the National Institutes of Health has not funded a single grant for either disease. The baleful consequence, as Marks points out, is the perpetuation of fallacies, myths, misconceptions, and anecdotal fictions regarding the pathogenesis and diagnosis, leading to confusions and controversies regarding treatment. He makes a valiant and successful effort to deal with these widespread misconceptions, which leave many patients neglected and undeserved. Marks stresses the enormous psychosocial impact these afflictions have on the quality of life, often leading to social isolation, depression, despair, loss of self-esteem, shame, anger, and even suicidal ideation. These diseases do not kill. Instead they can ruin life by limiting opportunities for all forms of life's societal interactions.

Marks is not only a prolific writer but is also highly esteemed for his ability to write plain, crystal-clear English, totally lacking in academic ostentatious, stuffy language.

This is an eminently readable and enjoyable text containing many memorable Marksian phraseologies; for example, his charge about the shameful lack of funding. He writes 'inflamed facial skin just cannot be ignored and always makes waves in the psychological stream'.

It is often said that by the time a text is published the material is already out of date. This dictum will not apply here. This book is a classic which will inform clinicians and investigators for decades to come because of its rich and vivid descriptions, abundant illustrations, trustworthy references, crisp summaries and figures, Throughout, Marks stresses the need to seek objective quantitative, verifiable data on all aspects of these varied diseases, replacing folklore with science.

The sections on treatment are laudable for their preciseness and conciseness among a monumental array of therapeutic options, which alone would necessitate a volume twice this size. The enormous pharmacologic and surgical interventions are tersely described and referenced.

This classic is perhaps the culminating achievement of Marks' long and distinguished career as a scholar, teacher, researcher, and clinician par excellence which history will surely designate as one of the most important and poignant figures of the latter half of 20th century dermatology.

Albert M Kligman MD PHD

Acknowledgments

Any enterprise of this kind needs the help and goodwill of many whose only rewards are the knowledge that they have been an important component of it and the gratitude of the author. Amongst this group I must pick out some for special thanks. My elder daughter, Louise, has with enormous skill and patience produced the manuscript from my scrawlings, even though we live about 150 miles from each other. My wife, Hilary, has given constant encouragement and helped in hundreds of ways. My gratitude also goes to Robert Peden of Informa Healthcare for this tolerance of my tardiness and help in the publication process. Thanks to you all – I hope you think that the final product is worth the effort.

Introduction

'My face is my fortune Sir she said.' The words of this traditional rhyme point to the central issue with facial rashes. The well-being of the human psyche and our self-regard seem dependent on what we perceive is an attractive facial appearance. A red rash on the most consistently exposed part of the human anatomy – the face – is extremely damaging to the way most of us feel about ourselves and if present for long periods, skin disorders causes a profound reactive depression.[1,2] Not unexpectedly there is some variability in the way that individuals respond to facial disorders of this sort with perhaps a greater depth of despair occurring in young women and an outwardly more disdainful and unconcerned attitude being found in older men. Even in this latter group, however, attitudes are changing and husky males now consult the mirror almost as often as young women. Make no mistake, visible skin disease of the face is disturbing to all who experience it however 'macho' we may think we are. Regardless of the particular social setting in which it occurs an inflamed or damaged facial skin just cannot be ignored and always makes waves in the psychological stream. The clinician must also be aware that some patients have a disturbed and distorted view of their skin leading them to complain bitterly about minor changes, which are hardly noticed by all others. This condition is known as dysmorphophobia and can be extremely difficult to deal with.[3]

Recognition and characterization of individual facial skin disorders has been sluggish compared to many other skin disorders. Rosacea was confused with acne for many years – and indeed still is by some authors. This relatively late recognition is one reason for the comparative ignorance of the nature of many common facial rashes. The lack of attention may also have been responsible for the comparatively little research on this topic.

Apart from the visibility of facial skin and the major impact that this has on the self-regard of the sufferer and on the views of peers what else is special about skin disease of this part of the anatomy which merits separate discussions?

Exposure to the vagaries and vicissitudes of the climate has an obvious major influence on the incidence, type and natural history of facial dermatoses. In particular, exposure to solar ultraviolet irradiation (UVR) is strongly implicated in or even solely responsible for causing some inflammatory skin disorders known as the photodermatoses and for localizing others to exposed areas of skin. Solar UVR is also responsible for causing the degenerative disorder known as solar elastotic degeneration, or as it is usually more simply referred to solar elastosis. This disorder is responsible for a constellation of physical signs which together form the major component of what has come to be known as photoaging – in fact it has little to do with aging itself. It is rather due to accumulated solar damage in exposed skin. Patchy brown spots and both non-melanoma and melanoma skin cancers, as well as their precursor lesions, are other problems caused by long continued sun exposure.

The chill wind, exposure to focal sources of heat and fluctuations in relative humidity are other climatic factors that almost certainly also play a role in modulating the condition of facial skin and in the expression of skin disease on the face.

Habitually exposed areas of skin are also more likely to encounter airborne and other allergens and irritants in the environment. Examples include allergic contact dermatitis to phosphorus sesquisulfide (found in some British red-headed matches) and flowers and plants such as chrysanthemums, primulae, poison ivy and certain kinds of moss. In addition any toxic or sensitizing external agents that the hands encounter are quite likely to be carried to the face and neck, a fact that should be remembered in trying to establish a diagnosis. The appearance of dermatitis near the eyes and on the sides of the neck in women who become sensitized to their nail cosmetics is a classic example of this.

Facial skin, then, is distinguished by being exposed to climatic influences and to chemical agents in the environment that can, in one way and another, harm it. It is also exposed to our prying and probing fingers which can do a surprising amount of harm. The lesions they cause vary from simple lichenification and pigmentation around the eyes in atopic dermatitis and the excoriated papule in the condition we know as acne excoreé to dramatically ulcerated areas in the hysterical disorder called dermatitis artefacta. The latter is often difficult to diagnose and is always difficult to treat.

To establish, confirm or refute the diagnosis of a facial skin disease there is no more valuable a procedure than skin biopsy. There is a natural reluctance to remove a small piece of facial skin but if performed with care and a few simple rules more is to be lost by not biopsying a facial rash than by performing the biopsy. The 'rules' are as follows:

- there should be no other way of reaching or confirming a diagnosis
- the procedure is unlikely to produce significant scarring (see later)
- the patient agrees and fully cooperates
- the histological section should be read by a pathologist with some experience of interpreting facial skin biopsies.

To minimize scarring, avoid sampling the nose and the paranasal areas if at all possible. Employ sharp disposable 4 mm 'punch' trephines and do not suture the small circular wound. The biopsy sites stop bleeding after a little firm pressure. If bleeding is persistent electrocautery may be used.

As might be expected facial skin also participates in generalized skin disorders such as erythroderma due to drug hypersensitivity, generalized seborrheic eczema, erythrodermic psoriasis, pityriasis rubra pilaris and T-cell lymphoma. Specific physical signs on facial skin develop in some systemic disorders and may be very helpful in reaching a definitive diagnosis.

The autoimmune (connective tissue) disorders, are, for example displayed in a characteristic way on the face. The swelling and the mauve bluish red (heliotrope) periocular discoloration and swelling seen in dermatomyositis is virtually pathognomonic of this disease. The well-known 'butterfly erythema' of the cheeks, in acute systemic lupus erythematosus, points stridently to the diagnosis of this multisystem disorder. A pinched 'beak-like' face, a small mouth that opens less wide than normal and with difficulty and telangiectatic macules over the cheek and nose are classical signs of systemic sclerosis. Other examples where observation of facial skin provides important clues to the diagnosis of a systemic illness include the suffusion and hirsutes on the upper cheeks in porphyria cutanea tarda and the severe seborrheic dermatitis seen in AIDS.

One other major reason for the special nature of facial rashes is that facial skin differs markedly from the skin of other regions in the detail of its anatomy. The profusion of pilosebaceous units with exaggeration of the sebaceous glands at some sites and the large terminal hairs at others also influences the expression of skin disease on the face. The large number of adnexal structures each surrounded by its own plexus of ramifying vascular elements disturbs the structural integrity of the dermal connective tissue and modulates its mechanical behavior. The mechanical response of facial skin to a physical stimulus must also be greatly influenced by the facial muscles in the subcutis as they have both dermal and deeper tissue attachments. The dermo–epidermal junction of facial skin tends to have a flattened profile with consequent reduction in prominence of the papillary dermis compared to limb or trunk skin. Most of the superficial capillary vasculature seems to reside in the prominent subpapillary venous plexus and inspection of a facial biopsy will confirm that papillary capillaries are poorly developed.

The prominence of pilosebaceous units with small hairs, but large sebaceous glands, the so-called 'acne follicles' and the flattened dermo–epidermal junction with a relatively thin epidermis, gives rise to the quite characteristic histological picture of facial skin.

There is no need for a special breed of dermatologist specializing in facial skin, but it is clinically worthwhile taking note of the special nature of facial skin and the disorders that affect it. What has been written above partially explains why facial dermatoses affect patients profoundly and why facial skin is prone to certain types of skin disease. It does not completely explain why some common skin disorders such as psoriasis and seborrheic dermatitis sometimes look quite different when they occur on facial skin and then frequently cause difficulty in diagnosis. The richness of the blood supply to facial skin and the nearness of the superficial vascular plexus to the skin surface and the ready dilation of its blood vessels, ensures that all inflammatory dermatoses affecting the face rapidly cause a deep erythema. It should also be remembered that the close proximity of several different types of skin with slightly differing characteristics (e.g. lips and perioral skin, nose and cheek skin) and facial contours may also help explain why facial rashes 'look different'.

Perhaps, not unexpectedly, there are special issues concerning the treatment of inflammatory dermatoses affecting the face. Thick greasy ointments are not appreciated and for similar cosmetic considerations colored topical preparations (e.g. tars) or those that stain should not be proffered; colorless lotions, thin creams, gels and mousses are usually preferred. Facial skin is easily irritated and many active agents such as the topical retinoids and vitamin D analogs should be prescribed cautiously and in lower concentrations than for limb and trunk skin. It is important to warn patients about the possibility of stinging, burning and irritation with these preparations; failure to do so is cause for justified complaint should an irritant response occur.

Corticosteroids are absorbed more easily through facial skin than through limb and trunk skin, and this is part of the reason that skin thinning occurs so readily on the face when potent topical corticosteroids are used. The telangiectasia and redness that this causes are the result of the ease with which the facial vasculature becomes dilated, and the 'loose weave' of the dermal connective tissue. Prescribing for facial skin requires some understanding of the potential problems, a little experience and a lot of humility.

References

1. Gupta MA, Gupta AK. Depression and suicide ideation in dermatology patients with acne, alopecia areata atopic dermatitis and psoriasis. Br J Dermatol 1998; 39: 846–9.
2. Sheerin D, MacLeod M, Kusumakar V. Psychological adjustment in children with port-wine stains and prominent ears. J Am Acad Child Adolesc Psychiatry 1995; 34: 1637–47.
3. Cotterill JA. Dermatologic nondisease Dermat Clin 1996; 14: 439–45.

Rosacea

Introduction

Rosacea is a common and cosmetically disabling disease which remains almost as mysterious now as when the disorder was first described. Despite its frequency and disfiguring nature it has provoked a relatively small amount of serious study. This is sad, as without a vigorous research effort new drugs will not emerge to treat the disease and our patients will remain dissatisfied with the treatments available. It is also quite inexplicable to me as it is such a fascinating disorder. It is fascinating because it consists of such diverse clinical features and tissue processes that are really quite difficult to link together. We can't even say with confidence that rosacea is just one disease and not several different disorders that have certain physical signs in common.

Part of the difficulty has been that authors have not always been too careful over the types of patient that they have grouped together as having rosacea in their study groups. Until recently no definitions of the disease have existed and without a universally accepted definition it is difficult to research or to teach about the condition. Few have addressed the issue of definition, the notable exception to this being the American National Rosacea Society Expert Committee.[1] As this latter group has pointed out 'the term rosacea has been applied to patients and research subjects with a diverse set of clinical findings that may or may not be an integral part of this disorder .... And there are no histologic or serologic markers'. The fact that there are no pathognomonic laboratory markers which can reliably identify the disorder is the central difficulty. The best that we can hope for is a histological report on a biopsy of a patient with a facial rash which says that the changes observed are 'consistent with rosacea' (see later). Nonetheless, we need to try to define the disorder in some way so that we can research it and learn more about it. At the present time we really have no choice but to define rosacea in clinical terms and to do this we need to use the physical signs, the sites of involvement as well as the chronology. The following then is the definition that I offer so that you, the reader, will know the type of patient to whom I refer. 'Rosacea is a common chronic persistent disorder of the skin of the face of unknown cause which is characterized by erythema and telangiectasia affecting the facial convexities and in particular the cheeks, the tip of the chin and forehead and the nose. Its course is punctuated by acute episodes of inflammation marked by intensification of the erythema, swelling papules and sometimes pustules.'

The essential component of the disease is the persistent erythema on the facial convexities and without this easily detectable sign the diagnosis must be considered suspect.

Some authors[2] see rosacea as a stepwise progression through several stages. They believe that the ready flushing and blushing often noted in this disease should be considered 'stage one' rosacea. An alternative and more attractive explanation to me is that the blushing is a consequence of the disorder and not a predisposing precursor and is by no means always seen right at the start of the condition.

Epidemiology

Virtually all who have written about rosacea seem to have agreed that the disease is most commonly seen in blue-eyed, fair-skinned North-Western European types. Individuals of Celtic ancestry seem especially prone and Powell and his Dublin colleagues have dubbed the disease 'the curse of the Celts'.[3] Informal enquiries amongst colleagues and my own clinical experience would tend to confirm that 'Celtic types' are quite often affected by rosacea. It is of interest to note that the Celts seem unduly prone to many sun-induced skin disorders including skin cancer.[4] Although rosacea seems to be very much more often a problem of the fair skinned it is by no means restricted to these. Rosacea is sometimes also seen in patients from the Mediterranean littoral, and in those from the Gulf States, from Asia Minor, from the Indian subcontinent and from South East Asia. There are also reports of the disease in Chinese and Japanese subjects. The only ethnic group in whom rosacea is extremely rare is black-skinned individuals of African extraction. Even this has been disputed in a report of ocular rosacea occurring in a group of black-skinned Americans.[5]

Regrettably there are few validated data concerning the occurrence of rosacea in any racial group and all of what has been said in the preceding paragraphs has the status of hearsay and anecdote rather than hard evidence-based fact. Until appropriate studies have been performed and published we have no choice but use what is available. One study worthy of mention from Scandinavia observed office workers returning from work and determined that some 10% had rosacea.[6] Despite the unusual methodology adopted in this study it certainly tends to confirm that rosacea is a common disease in north-west Europe!

It is usually said that rosacea is more common in women than in men. Certainly most 'series' of rosacea patients have more female than male patients within the group. The disease may indeed be more often a disease of women than of men but the increased proportion of women could also be due to unintentional bias. Women are reputed to care more about their facial appearance than do men (although the recent trend has been for this to be less noticeable) and this may well influence women to present to their doctors about a facial rash more readily than men. Perhaps men are also more reluctant to take time off work to see a physician for what they judge to be benign and trivial complaints – once again giving a false impression that rosacea is mostly a disease of women.

Rosacea is often said to be a disease of the mid-life years and, although there are no validated figures, experience suggests that the disease usually makes its first appearance between the ages of 25 and 55. Strangely the disorder appears to be less often seen in the 6th, 7th and later decades. Several reports have appeared of a rosacea-like disorder of infants.[7] Most of these unusual infants have developed their facial rash as a result of the use of topical corticosteroids – apparently even weak hydrocortisone-like over-the-counter steroid creams can be responsible.

No particular social class predisposition seems to exist. It has been suggested that workers exposed to a considerable amount of radiant heat such as cooks and boilermen are especially vulnerable to rosacea but once again there is only anecdotal evidence in favor of this intriguing possibility. It has also been said that rosacea is quite common in workers in the 'alcohol industry' such as barmen, vintners and brewery workers. Such limited study as there has been denies the relationship of alcohol with rosacea (see later).

Natural history

The disorder usually begins insidiously with the redness and telangiectasia gradually developing over some months. There are, however, some patients who do not seem to notice the increasing redness and whose first problem is an acute episode of papules and pustules accompanied by facial swelling. Such acute episodes usually settle within a few weeks with appropriate treatment (see later) or gradually subside over a much longer period. Complications such as rhinophyma or chronic lymphoedema are often remorselessly progressive. Long-term follow-up studies suggest that rosacea is indeed a very persistent disorder. Although acute episodes may remit so that very little in the way of visible abnormalities are then evident further attacks may develop some time later.[8,9]

History

Rosacea seems to have been recognized as a disorder long before dermatology became a separate branch of medicine. Clearly it was recognized in folklore and literature many years before any formal clinical description appeared. Chaucer's description[10] of the face of the 'pardoner' and Shakespeare's descriptions[11] of the convivial, lovable but quite naughty Falstaffian group make it plain that these authors knew the physical signs of rosacea. Rhinophyma – the distinctive nasal complication of rosacea – also appears in 'classical' painting.

Signs and symptoms

Sites affected

Rosacea is a chronic skin disorder confined to the face. It is true that in extremely rare instances lesions may develop outside of the face but such cases are indeed vanishingly rare and the opening statement of this section should remain our major clinical guideline. The areas of facial skin involved are almost exclusively the convexities so that the cheeks are affected up to the nasolabial folds (Figure 2.1). Nasal skin is often also affected so that there is 'butterfly' involvement of the two cheeks and the nose not dissimilar to the situation in systemic lupus erythematosus and erysipelas. The central area of the forehead is often involved. The erythema always stops at the hair line so that there is a striking contrast between the white scalp skin and the red of the rosaceous forehead skin. Similarly the skin of the eyebrow region is always spared. The upper lip is not affected by rosacea but the chin often is although the mental cleft is not. It will be noticed that the main areas of involvement – the cheeks, the forehead, the nose and the chin – are just those sun-exposed sites affected in the photodermatoses (see chapter 7).

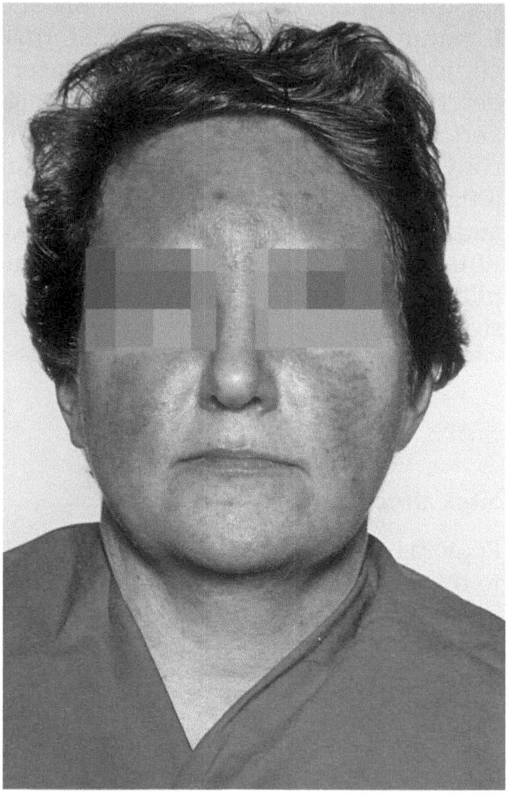

Figure 2.1

Early rosacea. Note that the facial convexities are affected – the cheeks, forehead, chin and nose show erythema and telangiectasia.

Unusual sites

Occasionally the front and sides of the neck develop signs of rosacea but this is quite uncommon. Periocular skin is not usually involved unless the complication of ocular rosacea develops (see below). In bald-headed men rosacea may develop on the exposed area of scalp skin[12] (Figure 2.2) – once again emphasizing

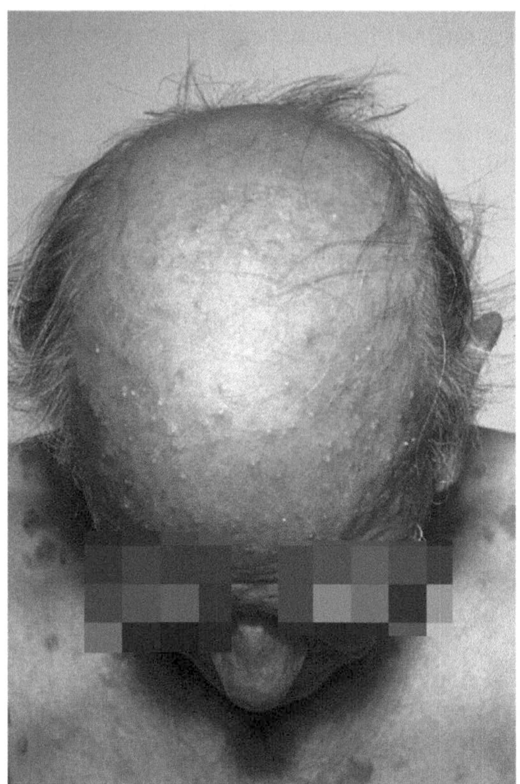

Figure 2.2

Rosacea of the bald scalp. The skin of the hair-bearing scalp is unaffected.

the distribution of the lesions on the convex light-exposed areas of the skin. The affected bald pate is reddened and studded with papules and sometimes pustules.

Uncommonly, signs of rosacea may develop asymmetrically over the face, involving one cheek more than the other (Figure 2.3). Rarely only one site is affected – such as one cheek. It is then extremely difficult to establish the diagnosis – requiring biopsy and the absence of evidence of any other disorder.

Rarely, lesions of rosacea have been reported to occur on sites outside of the head and neck.[13,14] However, there is some debate as to exactly how often this variant of rosacea is seen. One author[15] has stated that 15% of 53 patients with granulomatous rosacea had 'extra-facial' lesions but this report must be considered extremely unusual. The phenomenon of 'extra-facial' lesions is so uncommon that we need criteria before accepting that patients do indeed have 'disseminated' or 'extra-facial' rosacea. Clearly the first of these should be that the condition occurs during the course of an attack of straightforward facial rosacea. The second is that the lesions in the unusual sites bear some resemblance to those usually seen in ordinary facial rosacea: i.e. erythema, papules and pustules. The next important requirement is that the lesions are histologically compatible with rosacea. Finally, the peripheral lesions should not persist but should respond to treatment for rosacea and remit at approximately the same time as the facial disorder. It should be noted that in those cases in which it is reasonable to conclude that the condition seen was actually disseminated rosacea the lesions occurred in unexpected sites, such as grouped over the upper arms, wrists or knees. But the lesions themselves had no very special clinical features (Figure 2.4).

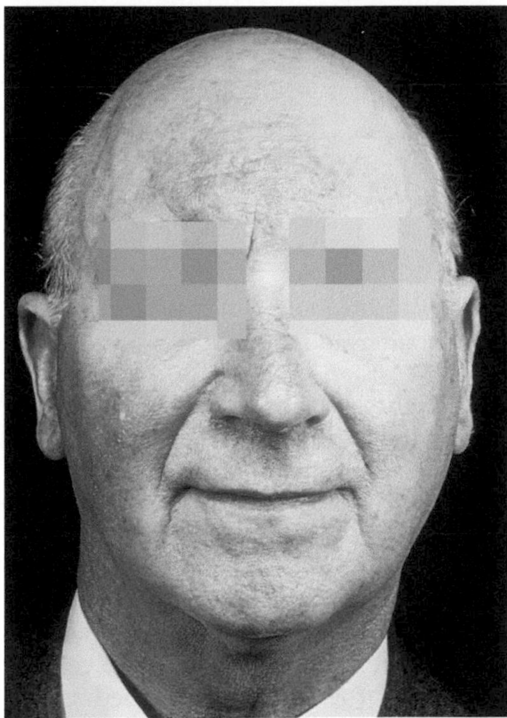

Figure 2.3

Rosacea with sparing of left cheek.

Lesions observed

Erythema/telangiectasia

The earliest sign of rosacea is persistent erythema affecting both cheeks symmetrically (Figure 2.5). The areas affected usually have poorly delineated borders. The erythema is often accompanied by a variable amount of telangiectasia which

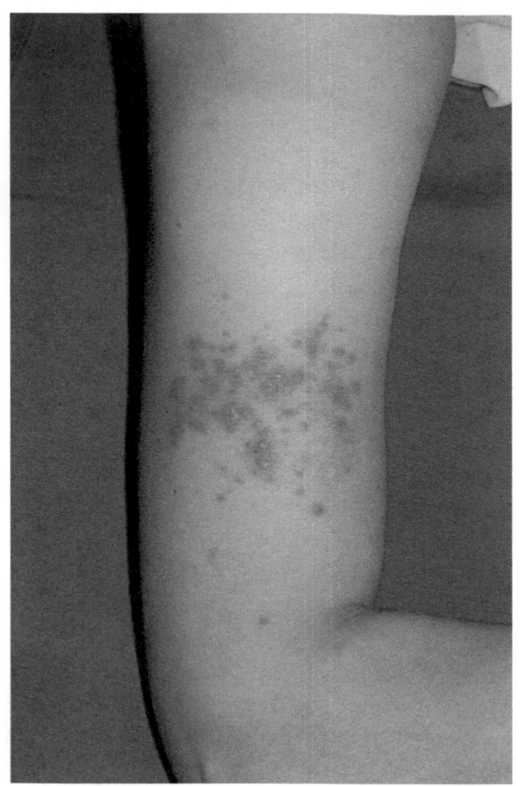

Figure 2.4

Disseminated (extra-facial rosacea). There is a cluster of red papules on the arm in a patient with typical rosacea of the face.

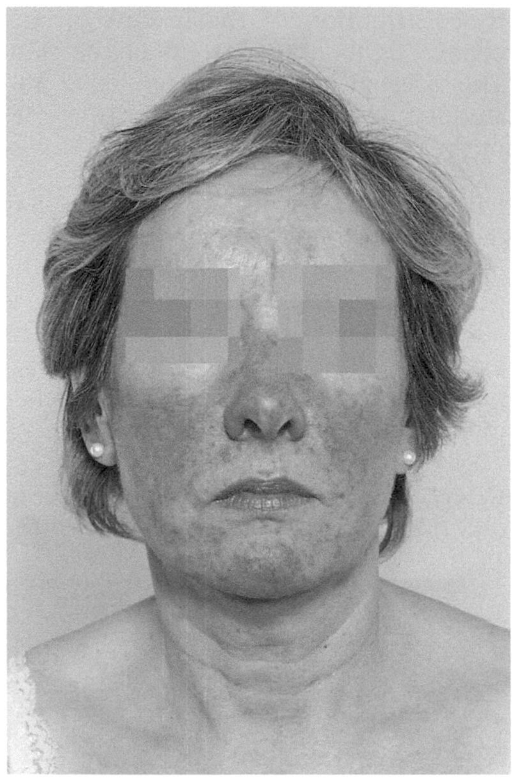

Figure 2.5

Typical distribution of rosacea on cheeks, chin, nose and forehead.

is best observed over the cheeks and nose and may be very marked in a few patients. Alongside the erythema is the complaint of flushing and blushing. This does not seem to occur in isolation but accompanying the erythema. Patients flush/blush more often, more deeply and more readily than do normal individuals.

The erythema is quite persistent and 'noticeable' and is much complained of by patients. Although persistent it may fluctuate in intensity and is often much influenced by the ambient temperature – the red cheeks tending to become mauve in the cold. This suggests that rather than there being an increased rate of blood flow in the affected skin the redness is due to pooling in the dilated superficial vasculature. In fact rosaceous cheeks do not feel hot as does an inflamed area of skin but feels quite cool to the touch. Borrie[16] measured the skin temperature of the erythematous areas and found that it was in the normal range.

Alongside the erythema there is often a network of variously sized small blood vessels – telangiectasia – known popularly, for some curious reason as 'broken veins'. They are often a source of great embarrassment. The longer the disease has been present the more prominent is the telangiectasia.

Papules and pustules

These lesions arise suddenly without any obvious provocation and vary greatly in number. During a severe attack there is often marked accompanying oedema. Indeed, some degree of facial swelling is often seen in rosacea – even when non-inflamed. The papules are usually pink or light red in color and hemispherical in shape (Figure 2.6). They are neither tender nor painful unlike the papules in acne. They do not arise around poral orifices and, interestingly, they all appear at the same stage of development. Pustules occur less commonly in rosacea than in acne – being seen in perhaps 10% of patients.

Differential diagnosis

The main common differential diagnoses to consider are acne, seborrheic dermatitis and perioral dermatitis. Table 2.1 summarizes the main features that distinguish these disorders.

Regrettably, the disease is not always as easy to differentiate as it should be theoretically. For example, in severe facial acne the persistent severe inflammation may result in a degree of background redness which can be confused with rosacea – a situation that can be referred to as 'red acne' (Figure 2.7). Also some topical medications cause minor irritation and scaling so that the condition can be mistaken for an eczematous disorder. Also because all the differential diagnoses mentioned are quite common occasionally two of the diseases may coexist – without there being any special or significant relationship between the disorders.

Photosensitivity disorders cause eczematous rashes in light-exposed sites so that

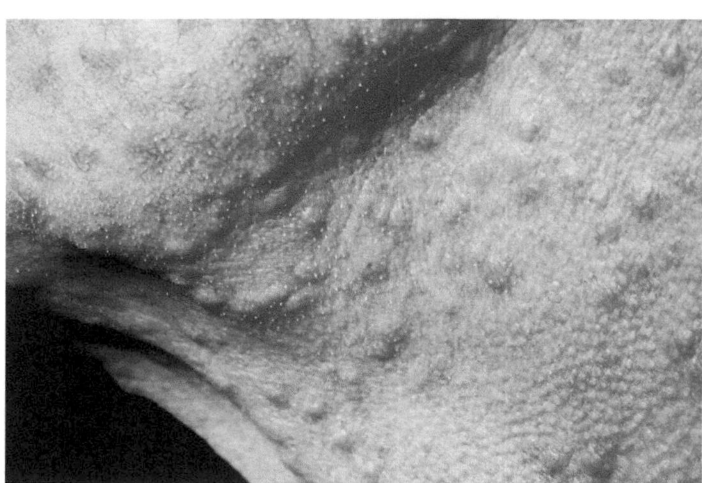

Figure 2.6

Typical rosacea papules – pink, hemispherical and non-tender.

TABLE 2.1 Main distinguishing features of common differential diagnoses

CLINICAL FEATURE	ROSACEA	ACNE	SEBORRHEIC DERMATITIS	PERIORAL DERMATITIS
Background of erythema	Yes – marked	Not usually	Some but variable	Minimal
Telangiectasia	Yes	None	None	None
Seborrhea	None	Yes – maybe marked	Not obvious	None
Papules	Yes – non-tender pink hemispherical	Irregular – tender	None	Yes – micropapules
Cysts	None	Sometimes	None	None
Scars	None	Often	None	None
Sites involved	Face – alone	Face, shoulders, back, chest	Facial flexures, scalp, body flexures	Perioral

similar areas to those in rosacea are affected on the face. However, the involvement of other light-exposed areas such as the backs of the hands and the 'V' of the neck as well as the classical eczematous changes seen in photosensitivity should distinguish this group of disorders from rosacea.

Rosacea may also be confused with the facial rash of erysipelas as the swollen red eruption of this disorder may be symmetrical involving either cheek (Figure 2.8). The fever, the malaise, the sudden onset, the tenderness, the well-defined (and sometimes hemorrhagic) edge as well as the rapid response to penicillin should all serve to distinguish this condition.

Systemic lupus erythematosus may cause the well-known and distinctive butterfly rash which affects either cheek and the bridge of the nose (Figure 2.9), but there is usually no difficulty in differentiating this disorder from rosacea because of the rash elsewhere and the accompanying systemic complaints and the various laboratory abnormalities. Discoid lupus erythematosus causes irregular, asymmetrical scarring plaques and is not difficult to tell apart from rosacea but there is a quite rare variant of LE known as papular LE in which the main feature is the appearance of facial papules. These can closely simulate the papules of rosacea save there is not the background of erythema (Figure 2.10). Skin biopsy will easily distinguish all forms of LE from rosacea.

Dermatomyositis is another of the autoimmune disorders whose skin signs can be confused with rosacea. Typically the condition involves the upper face – particularly

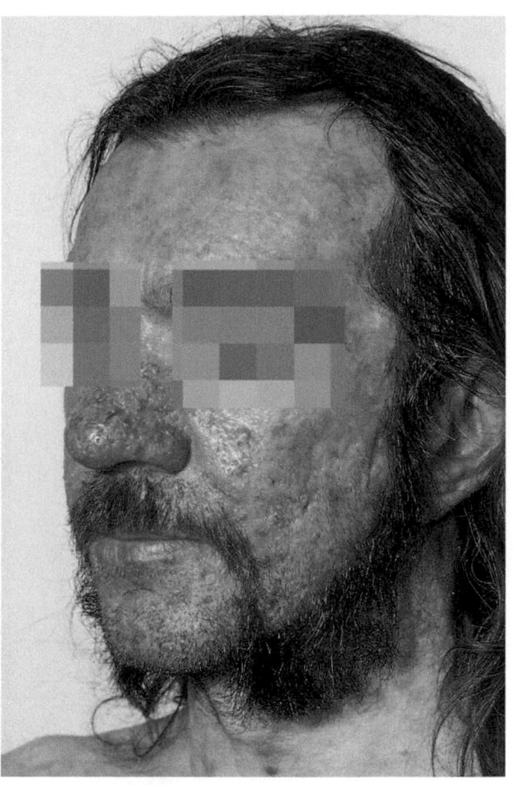

Figure 2.7

'Red acne'. This young man has acne – note the greasy appearance of the skin and the scarring.

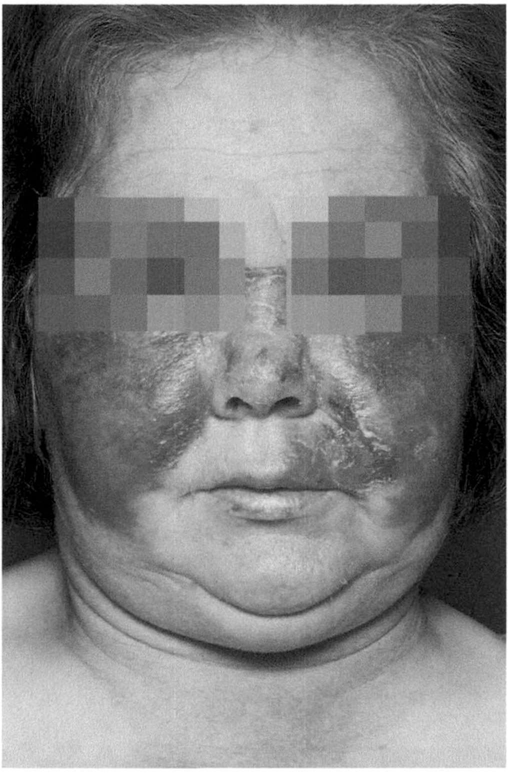

Figure 2.8

Erysipelas. The reddened area is in the butterfly distribution.

the periocular tissues – causing swelling and a mauve–lilac (heliotrope) discoloration. Mostly such patients have signs of muscle disease also, including weakness and tenderness in addition to the characteristic laboratory findings of inflammation, and muscle disease. Other systemic disorders may occasionally simulate rosacea – including polycythemia rubra vera in which the entire face may become suffused and plethoric. Also, superior vena cava obstruction may cause the face to become swollen and suffused with dilated veins in the neck and over the upper chest. In the carcinoid syndrome a bowel tumor of the argentaffin cells metastasizes to the liver and secretes 5-hydroxytryptamine causing intermittent flushing, facial telangiectasia and very rarely a rosacea-like disorder.

Variants and complications

Variants in which unusual sites are involved (scalp, disseminated, asymmetrical facial) have already been described (see page 8).

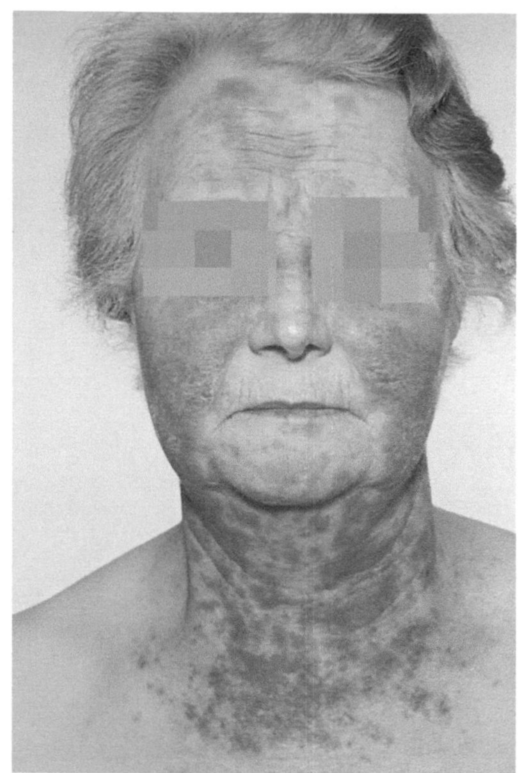

Figure 2.9

This lady had systemic lupus erythematosus. Note the patchy erythematous plaques over the face and neck.

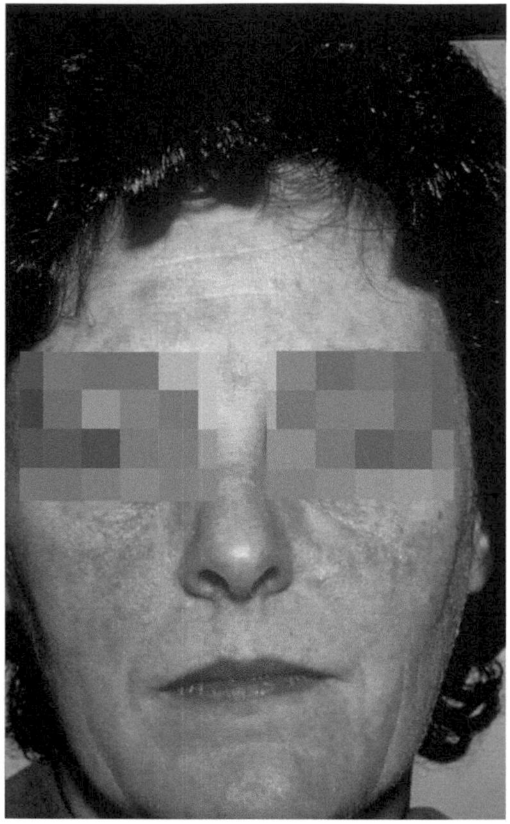

Figure 2.10

Papular LE. The clinical appearance can closely simulate rosacea.

Rhinophyma

This odd disorder is mainly an accompaniment of longstanding rosacea but also occurs rarely as an isolated phenomenon and very rarely as a complication of severe acne. When complicating rosacea, there is no relationship between the severity of the condition and the development of rhinopyhma. For some curious reason it is largely restricted to men (perhaps less than 10% are women). Clinically the disorder causes irregular thickening of the nose (Figure 2.11). There is prominence and dilatation of the pilosebaceous poral orifices and the entire nose is irregularly discolored all shades of red and mauve giving a distinctive if somewhat grotesque appearance (Figure 2.11).

Quite uncommonly other facial sites may be involved by the same process – the chin, the ear lobes and the adjoining cheeks

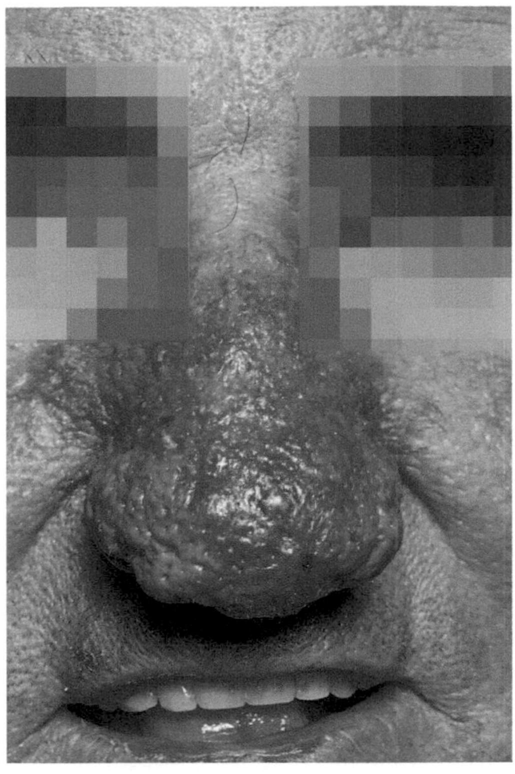

Figure 2.11

Nasal reddening and irregular swelling in rhinophyma.

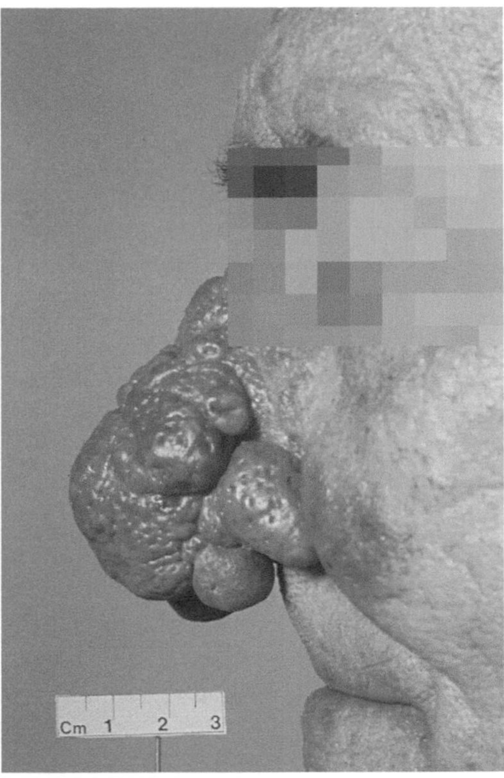

Figure 2.11a

Severe rhinophyma.

being occasionally affected in this way. The condition is slowly progressive and although it clearly causes tremendous cosmetic disability, some patients only present after the condition has been present for many years. The disorder has become associated in the public mind with alcoholism – for which there is no good evidence and folk names such as 'whiskey nose', or 'grog blossom' abound. In fact when specifically sought no relationship between rhinophyma and alcoholism has been found.[17]

Lymphoedema

Men are also the main sufferers of this odd complication of rosacea – persistent lymphoedema of facial tissues. There is some slight swelling of facial skin in many patients with rosacea ordinarily but this is mostly transient and slight in degree. In persistent lymphoedema the swelling is localized to a particular area – the periocular site being the one usually affected (Figure 2.12). The swelling is quite recalcitrant and apart from minor

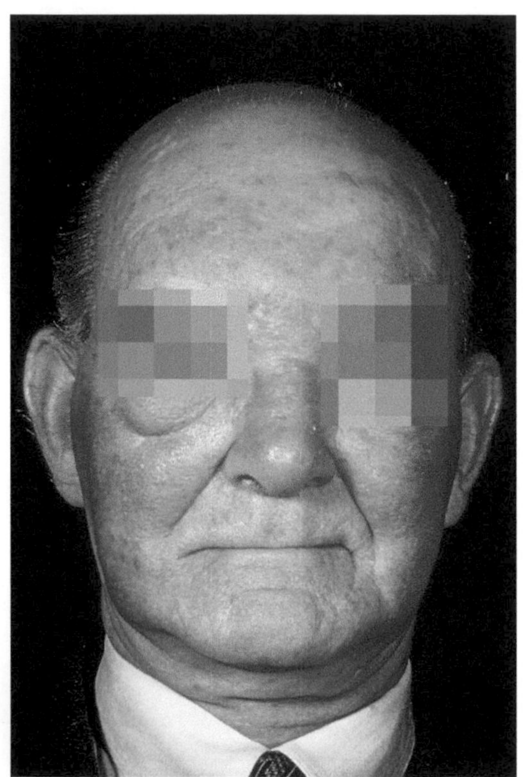

Figure 2.12

Persistent lymphoedema – most marked in the left periocular region.

fluctuations it does not alter in appearance over many months. Surgical 'debulking' procedures have been more successful than any other form of treatment.[18]

Ophthalmological complications

One of the greatest mysteries surrounding rosacea is the involvement of the eyes. It is not as if there were just one type of ocular involvement – there are several. The commonest eye problem experienced by rosacea patients is conjunctivitis. Some 20–30% of patients with acute papular rosacea develop blepharoconjunctivitis while a few also develop inflammation of the uveal tract. Alongside the marginal blepharitis styes, meibomian gland inflammation and tiny cysts (chalazion) are also seen. Perhaps even more difficult to explain is the keratoconjunctivitis sicca that some 30% of patients develop[19] – certainly when a Schirmer test is performed on patients with rosacea a surprisingly large number give a positive result. All the above ocular disorders give rise to discomfort and pain and may temporarily interfere with vision – but they are all transient and remit when the rosacea quietens or the condition is treated.

There is one ophthalmological complication, however, that is seriously disabling, very painful and that can produce permanent visual impairment. This is rosaceous keratitis. Curiously, as with rhinophyma and lymphoedema, it is a complication virtually exclusive to men but fortunately it is quite rare. The condition starts with severe pain in the eye and on examination a vascular pannus can be seen at the edge of the iris edging onto the cornea. This inflammatory pannus is destructive and causes corneal scarring. It tends to be remittent over long periods and may require corneal grafting to restore vision.

Pathology

Clinicians are for the most part reluctant to biopsy facial skin to confirm the diagnosis of a benign disease. Their reluctance to do so accounts for the comparative lack of experience of most dermatopathologists at seeing the various types and stages of rosacea down a microscope and consequently the quite cautious reports they usually issue when confronted by such a specimen. In fact providing due care is taken, biopsy of facial skin is rarely the cause of discernible scarring or other complication. My experience is that a 3 or 4 mm diameter punch biopsy does not require suturing – these small wounds heal better with very little scarring when no sutures are inserted. The site selected is also important as the nose, paranasal areas and adjoining cheeks seem to scar noticeably more often than do other areas.

Early rosacea

Erythematotelangiectatic rosacea is infrequently biopsied but when it is the changes observed are quite similar to those seen in what is sometimes called 'weathering'. The disruption of the usual architecture of the upper dermis is striking, the dermal connective tissue appears fragmented and disoriented. The disturbance of the dermis is compounded by the loss of the papillary structure with diminution of the rete pattern and by the presence of a variable amount of solar elastotic degenerative change (Figure 2.13). Set in the midst of this fragmented and distorted dermis are many irregularly dilated vascular channels (Figure 2.14). For the most part these are empty of blood, provoking the speculation that they are in fact lymphatic in origin. These vessels are often surrounded by a space, although we have also observed that there is thickening and an increase in connective tissue around a few of the vessels[20] (Figure 2.15). There are a few scattered mononuclear cells present, which tend to be clustered around the dilated vessels though not closely applied to the vessel as in discoid lupus erythematosus (Figure 2.16).

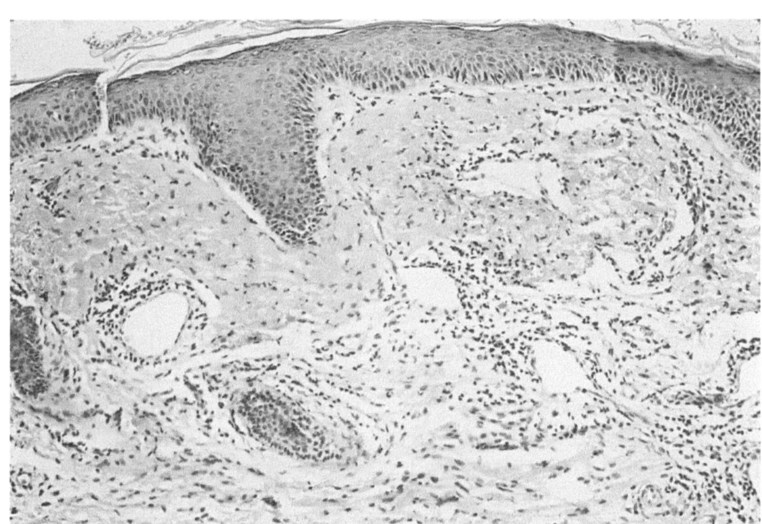

Figure 2.13

The histological picture in erythematotelangiectatic rosacea showing loss of the normal fibrillary structure of the dermis and multiple dilated vessels (hematoxylin and eosin × 45).

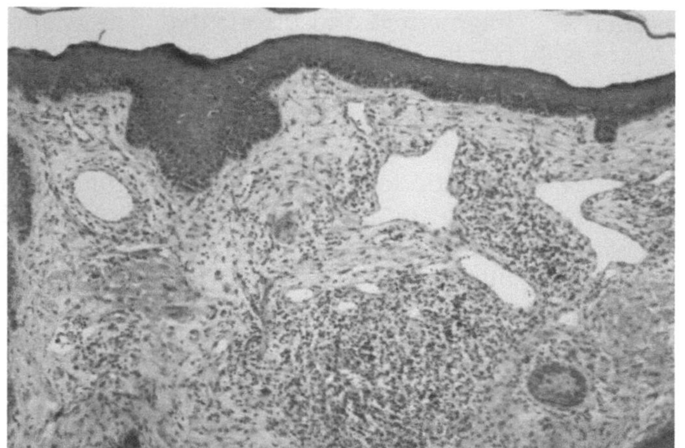

Figure 2.14

This histological picture is similar to Fig 2.13 save that there is a marked mononuclear inflammatory cell infiltrate around the widely dilated vascular spacers (hematoxylin and eosin × 45).

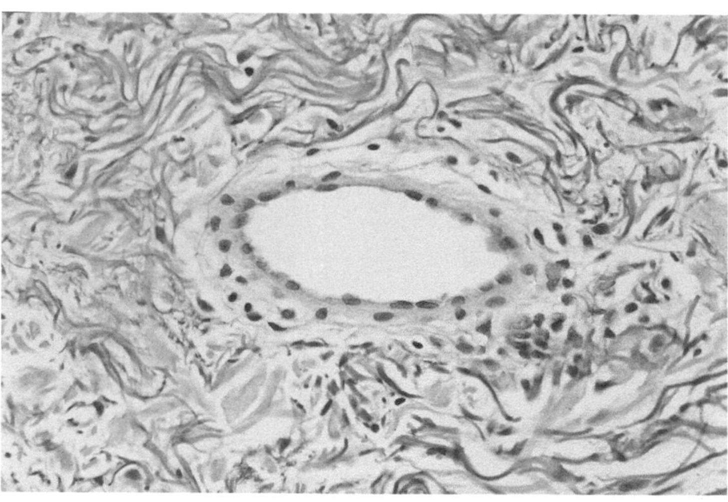

Figure 2.15

Some of the dilated vessels in the dermis have thickened walls. (hematoxylin and eosin × 150).

Inflammatory rosacea

The dermal dystrophy described above is evident in all samples examined. In addition to the background of fragmented and wan dermal connective tissue there is usually a degree of oedema. 'Inflammatory' cells are always much in evidence in this stage of the disease – they are mononuclear in type although a very small number of polymorphonuclear cells are sometimes also present. In addition and amongst the denser collections of inflammatory cells there are larger epithelioid mononuclear cells and maybe some giant cells (Figure 2.16) – approximately 10% of biopsies from inflamed papules contain giant cells. These are of the foreign body type although no particular material can be seen within these cells. Despite the belief of some authors that the inflammatory change stems from

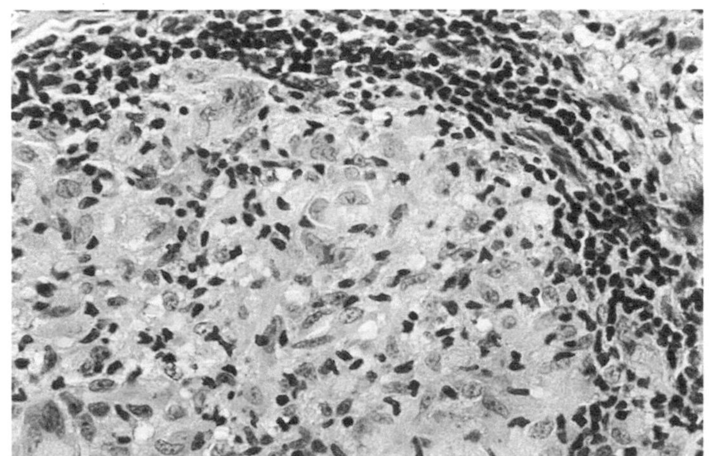

Figure 2.16

Epithelioid cells and giant cells are often seen as part of the granulomatous inflammation in inflammatory rosacea (hematoxylin and eosin × 150).

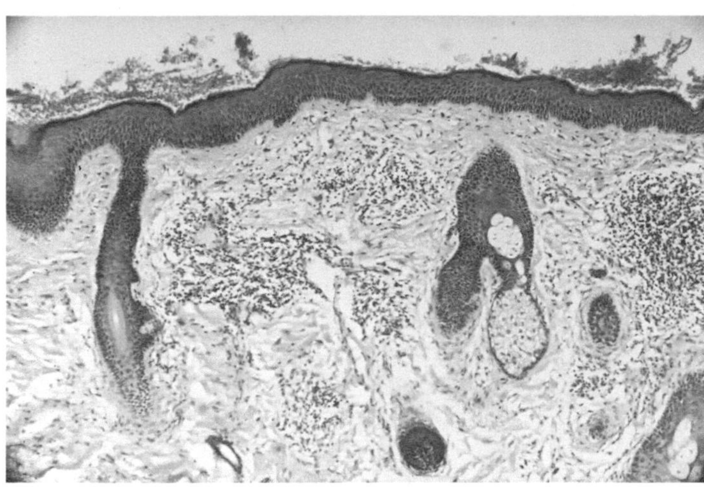

Figure 2.17

The inflammation is predominantly perivascular rather than around follicles (hematoxylin and eosin × 45).

the pilosebaceous structures there is no real evidence in favor of this. Horizontal, oblique and serial sections through blocks have failed to identify a follicular abnormality to account for the inflammation.[21] In fact inflammatory cells are mostly found around the vessels in the mid dermis rather than involving the follicles (Figure 2.17). When inflammatory cells seem to surround a follicle it is likely that they are there because of the rich vasculature around the follicles rather than because of any abnormality of the follicles themselves. One major reason for the suspicion that the follicles are in some way involved stems from the observation that there is an increased population of hair follicle mites (*Demodex folliculorum*) in rosacea (Figures 2.18 and 2.18a). Several groups have reported the very large numbers of these minute creatures (0.1 mm in length)[22,23] living in the facial follicles of rosacea patients compared to control groups, but as yet no evidence

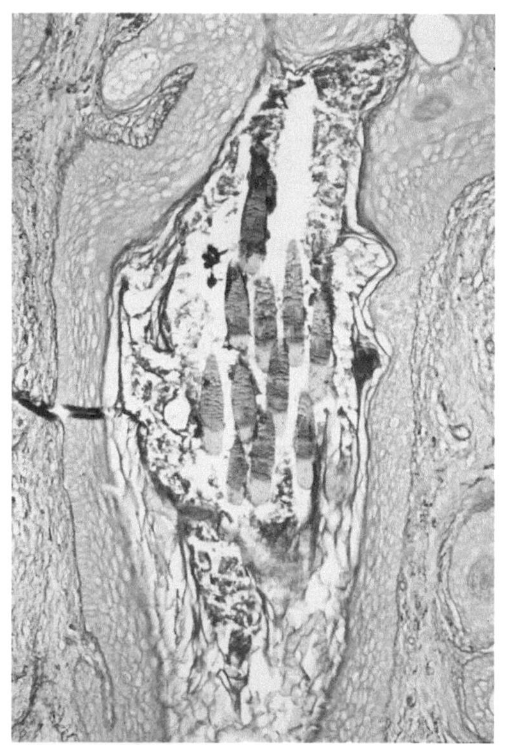

Figure 2.18

There are many *Demodex folliculorum* mites packed into this follicle (haematoxylin and eosin × 150).

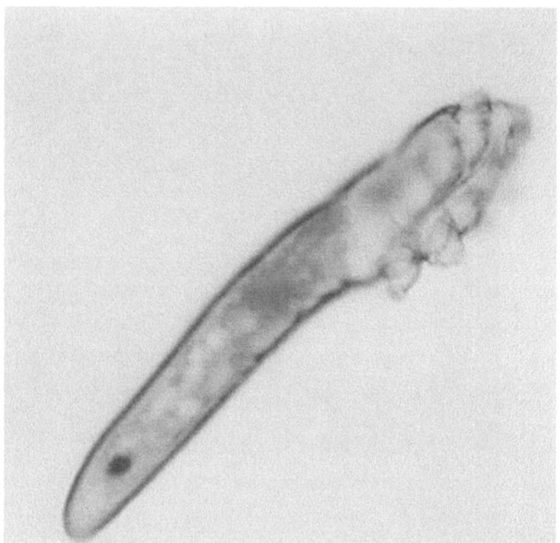

Figure 2.18a

Demodex folliculorum (× 250).

has been produced to suggest that they have a causative role. It is true that there have been rare reports of the demodex mite being found at the center of granulomata – but mostly the mites seem to live as harmless commensals in the follicles. A condition of papular demodicidosis has also been described[24] but the criteria for distinguishing this disorder are not clear. Similarly its possible relationship to rosacea is still a matter for discussion.

Rhinophyma

Once again there is a marked dermal dystrophy in the upper dermis accompanied by marked telangiectasia. There are often many inflammatory cells – mostly mononuclears but also polymorphs are present (Figure 2.19). There is also striking sebaceous gland hyperplasia with the enlarged lobules placed very near the skin surface. In many specimens there are also many fibrocytes throughout the sample and new collagenous strands coursing through the dermis.

The cause and pathogenesis of rosacea

It has been tacitly assumed in the past that there is but one cause of rosacea. It should be recognized however, that this

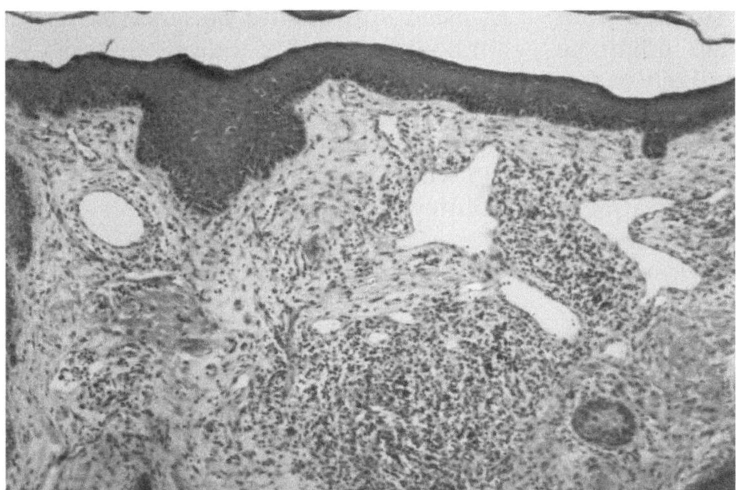

Figure 2.19

There is marked telangiectasia and a marked inflammatory cell infiltrate in this biopsy from rhinophyma (hematoxylin and eoxin × 45).

is not necessarily the case and that what we see in a patient with the physical signs of rosacea is the final common pathway of one of a number of different processes most of which are unrecognizable. It seems probable to the writer that there are indeed many causes but there is one major cause accounting for the majority of patients that we see.

Historically there has been a profusion of suggestions as to what is the underlying cause of this disease. They have embraced a wide variety of possible agencies but for the most part have not been supported by credible evidence. In the period around the middle of the last century the literature on the topic was elegant, imaginative but confusing, leaving one with the impression that rosacea was either a psychiatric disorder, the result of gastrointestinal dysfunction or conceivably a dietary problem.

The literature concerning a psychiatric cause often suggested that the flushing that occurs in rosacea is the result of guilt or some other deep emotional disturbance.[25] Any psychological disturbance in rosacea patients is in my view more likely to be the result of the appearance of the disease rather than the cause. When tested with a STENS personality inventory questionnaire, rosacea patients were found to be more depressed than matched controls[26] and this was interpreted as the result of the disease. It was thought to be expected in any persistent and difficult to remove skin disorder of the face. There are patients who are greatly disturbed at any minor blemish of facial skin – including a minor degree of facial reddening. The disorder of these individuals is often barely visible to onlookers – indeed the 'reddening' may exist only in the mind of the patient. Such patients are said to have dysmorphophobia[27] and can be extremely challenging to manage – particularly as the patients insist that they are suffering from rosacea.

There is also an extensive literature on suggestions that there is a gastrointestinal cause of rosacea. At first it was claimed that patients with rosacea suffered from indigestion more often than might be expected and that they were likely to suffer from hypochlorhydria.[28] On the basis of this belief patients were prescribed large amounts of dilute hydrochloric acid. As no controlled clinical trials of this treatment were reported then or since it cannot be said whether this relatively innocuous treatment produced any benefit. As subsequent studies have not succeeded in identifying any gastrointestinal abnormality in rosacea[29] the treatment seems to have been based on a false premise and without evidence of efficacy the practice has gone out of fashion. At one point the claim was made that rosacea patients suffered from malabsorption[30] but the study was not adequately controlled and later it was found that a control population had as many small bowel abnormalities as rosacea patients.[31] Interestingly in more recent times there have been several reports of 'infection' of rosacea patients with the micro-organism responsible for peptic ulceration – *Helicobacter pylori*.[32,33] Tests based on the metabolic activity of *H. pylori* and on the presence of serum antibodies seemed to indicate that rosacea patients were infected. However, further studies have not succeeded in incriminating this bacterium and it seems that it too will be cast into the dustbin of gastrointestinal hypotheses.[34]

It ought to be added that no other bacterial pathogen has been identified as playing a role in the pathogenesis of rosacea. Some have believed that the demodex mite is involved in the pathogenesis of this disease and this idea receives some support from the greatly increased numbers of demodices in rosacea.[35,36] As discussed above the evidence for this is somewhat slim. Although the follicles may be packed with demodex mites the follicles are not in fact the focal points of inflammation (see page 19). There have been some reports of parts of the mite being found in the middle of inflammatory foci[37] but it should also be pointed out that the mite is occasionally seen sitting in the middle of skin tissue without any surrounding inflammation (Figure 2.20).

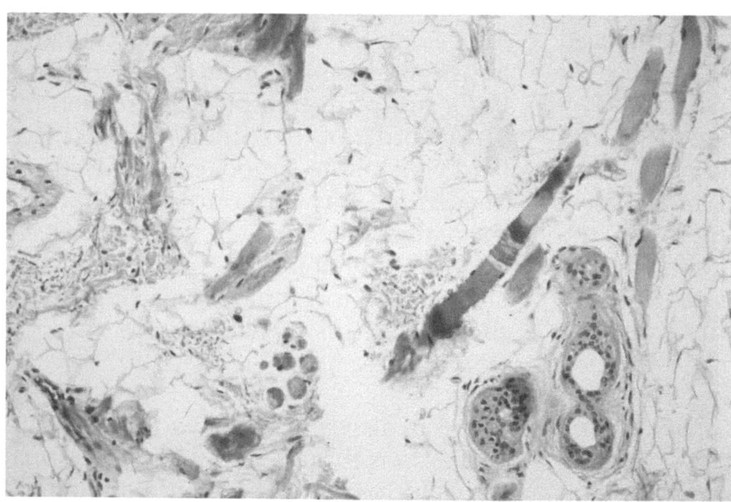

Figure 2.20

A demodex mite is present in the dermis without any inflammation (hematoxylin and eosin × 150).

Few of the successful therapeutic agents for rosacea are directly miticidal. However, sulfur, ivermectin and lindane have all been used to treat rosacea patients and have been shown to be able to kill mites. Whether any clinical improvement seen is due to an effect on mites is another issue. It is possible, of course, that the increase in mites could be a result of rosacea rather than being the cause. The dilated follicles in rosacea and the dilatation of the superficial capillary vasculature with pooling of the blood might well provide an attractive microclimate for the demodices.

Having said what does not appear to be the cause of rosacea, is there a candidate left worthy of serious consideration? The occurrence of rosacea on sun-exposed areas of facial skin and its predilection for fair-skinned, poorly pigmented subjects have led to the suggestion that photo damage may play a role in its development. Furthermore, histological studies reveal the presence of a significant amount of solar elastotic degenerative change[21] (Figure 2.21). Alongside the elastosis the upper dermis appears edematous and to have lost its usual fibrillar structure, assuming a disorganized and dystrophic appearance. Little is known about the cause of this dermal dystrophy, although it may well also be climatically induced. Anyway, the pronounced solar elastosis and the clinical clues mentioned above favor the disorder being photoinduced in some way – at least in part.

The consequences of the dermal disorganization are that the connective tissue framework fails to support the capillaries in the upper dermis; these then passively dilate. The pooling of the blood in these dilated vessels may be an important component of the pathogenesis as in their 'low-flow' hemodynamic state the endothelium of these dilated vessels may become hypoxic and leaky. They may then allow inflammatory macromolecules to diffuse into the dermis and cause inflammation. Figure 2.21a is a schematic summarizing this hypothetical pathogenetic sequence. Conclusive evidence for this view

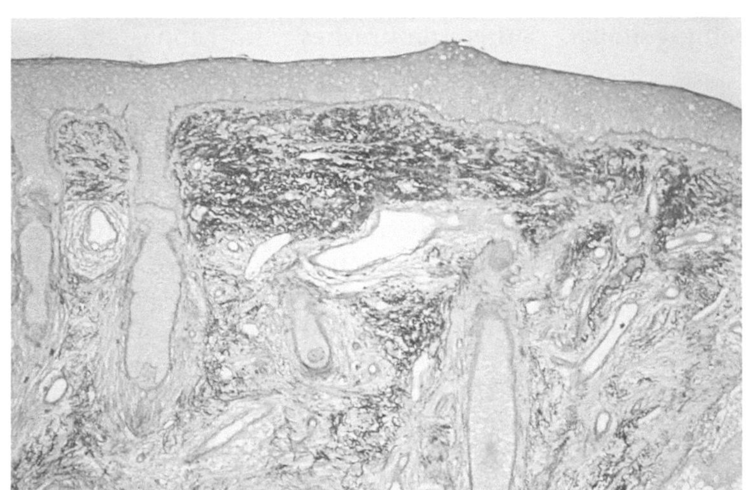

Figure 2.21

There is a mauve staining band subepidermally due to solar elastotic degeneration in rosacea (Halmi elastic stain × 45).

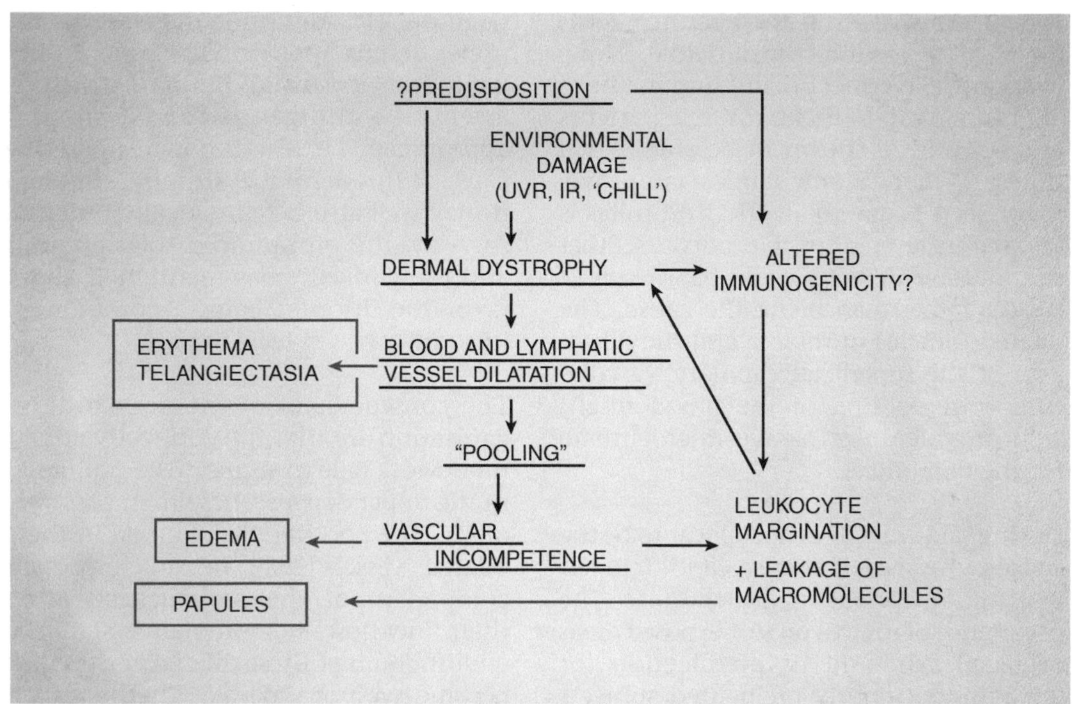

Figure 2.21a

Algorithm showing a possible sequence of events in the pathogenesis of rosacea.

does not yet exist but it seems that most clinical and histological observations can be explained by this or something similar.

The management of rosacea

General measures

Rosacea is a distressing and cosmetically disabling disorder and many patients become quite depressed. It should go without saying that such patients should be handled sensitively and sympathetically. Some patients benefit by consulting a cosmetician with camouflaging skills. Foundation creams and other 'leave-on' cosmetics should be completely non-irritating and if possible green tinted as this diminishes the appearance of redness.

Many patients with rosacea are made worse by sun exposure and advice concerning sun avoidance or at least how to minimize exposure should be proffered. Sunscreens which block both long-wave (UVA) and medium-wave (UVB) ultraviolet radiation should also be advised. Avoiding hot and spicy foods seems to do little – other than to make life a little more dull for the unfortunate patients. There is no doubt, however, that some patients flush markedly with certain foods and alcohol. There is no evidence of improvement if they go on an avoidance diet but some patients appreciate the reduction of flushing.

Rosacea patients often have very sensitive skin and emollient application and cleansing agents soothe the hot sore skin and give considerable relief. There is one other piece of general advice concerning topical applications – *topical corticosteroids must not be used.* These powerful agents do reduce the inflammatory papules but at the same time they make the skin redder and more telangiectatic. The redness persists even when the steroids are stopped. The cause of this paradoxical reddening is the skin-thinning effect of topical corticosteroids. The already dystrophic dermal connective tissue is made even more weak and inefficient by the use of the steroids, causing even further passive capillary dilation and further reddening.

Topical therapy

Topical metronidazole was one of the earliest active agents to be used for rosacea. It is formulated as a 0.75% or 1.0% gel or cream. In trials it reduced the number of inflammatory papules progressively after 3 weeks of use till at 9 weeks there was a 65% reduction of papules in one study[38] and a 75% reduction in another.[39] In comparative studies metronidazole was found to be as effective as oral oxytetracycline[39,40] and as effective as 20% azelaic acid[41] (see later). It causes drying and stinging in a few patients. Its mode of action is unknown.

Azelaic acid (15 or 20%) has been shown to be a safe and effective treatment for rosacea. Double-blind studies[42] demonstrated that 15% azelaic acid gel significantly reduced the inflammatory lesions and the erythema in patients with papulopustular rosacea within 4–8 weeks.[43,44] It is suggested that this material is effective in reducing the erythema. It certainly has been shown to be as effective as topical metronidazole as a therapeutic agent[45] and to be well accepted by patients without any significant adverse side effects. Its mode of action is unknown.

Various other agents have been claimed as effective topical medications – including a combination cream of 10% sulfacetamide and 5% sulfur. This has been shown in a double-blind vehicle-controlled study[46] and a topical metronidazole controlled study[47] to be safe and effective in papulopustular rosacea. In fact the combination of sulfur and sulfacetamide was found to be significantly more effective than the metronidazole at 12 weeks (80% compared to 72%).

How any of the topical agents discussed above work is quite mysterious but at least there is some rationale to the use of topical retinoids in rosacea. Granted that photo damage may be playing some role in the pathogenesis of the disease then the anti-photo damage action of the retinoids might be expected to be useful in rosacea. It has been claimed that topical tretinoin,[48] topical retinaldehyde[49] and topical adapalene[50] have useful therapeutic effects in rosacea. Personal experience has confirmed their usefulness in some patients. Regrettably, the irritant effects of the retinoids preclude their use for most rosacea patients.

The systemic action (see later) of the antibiotics and the anti-inflammatory activity of the antibiotics has suggested that these agents may have a role when applied topically. But there have been few credible reports of a useful action of topical antibiotics in rosacea although clindamycin phosphate (1%)[51] was reported as having a useful therapeutic effect. In an open study erythromycin and 2% azithromycin were thought to reduce the number of lesions.[52]

Both tacrolimus (0.075%)[53] and pimecrolimus (1%)[54] have been reported as helpful in patients with erythematotelangiectatic rosacea – the former specifically for patients with steroid-induced rosacea.

Topical 4-ethoxybenzaldehyde (4%) is a prototypic anti-inflammatory agent that has been trialed in rosacea. It was found to significantly reduce the erythema compared to placebo applied topically.[55]

Ivermectin has been employed as an oral anti-onchocercal agent in onchocerciasis for many years. It has also been employed in scabies as it has a miticidal action too. Because of these actions a topical preparation has been used and found effective in papular rosacea. Recently, because of a supposed demodicidal action, permethrin has been tried in inflammatory rosacea and found to be quite effective.[56]

Laser therapy

Pulsed tunable dye laser and pulsed high-energy light have both been claimed as successful modalities for reduction of the redness of rosacea. After up to three treatments each separated by 2–3 weeks not only has the redness and telangiectasia decreased but the inflammatory papules have also been found to decrease.[57–59]

Photodynamic therapy has also been used and claimed to be successful.

Oral treatments

The tetracyclines are of considerable dermatological interest as they have so many useful biochemical actions and resulting therapeutic effects.[60] They are known to reduce protein synthesis by an action on ribosomes as well as reduce neoangiogenesis, proteolysis, apoptosis and neutrophil bullous disorders,[61,62] pyoderma gangrenosum and pustular disorders.[47]

The various tetracyclines provide a reliably effective, safe and acceptable form of treatment for most patients with papular rosacea. Tetracycline itself is quite satisfactory giving an 80% reduction in lesions at 6 weeks,[63] but mostly the low-dose tetracycline agents are employed as they are certainly as, if not more, effective than the older agents and can be given either daily or twice daily and independently of meals. My personal favorite is doxycycline as it is associated with a low risk of adverse side effects compared to minocycline.[64] All tetracycline agents do, however, have a significant risk of teratogenicity for the pregnant woman and alternative treatments must be used. An anti-inflammatory dose of doxcycline 40 mg (30 mg immediate-release, 10 mg delayed-release beads) is supported by two randomized, placebo-controlled, multicentered, double-blind, 16-week studies involving 537 patients with rosacea. The drug provided a statistically significant reduction in inflammatory lesions (papules and pustules). The adverse reactions seen in the treatment group were comparable to placebo. No photosensitivity or vaginal candidiasis were seen in the treatment group. Interestingly, in vivo microbiological studies for up to 18 months demonstrated no detectable long-term effects on bacterial flora of the oral cavity, skin, intestinal tract and vagina. This finding may suggest that the efficacy of doxycyline in the treatment of rosacea may be attributed to its ability to suppress inflammatory mediators, rather than to its antimicrobial properties.

In the clinical trial of tetracycline mentioned above – comparisons were made both with placebo and with ampicillin. Ampicillin was found to be significantly more effective than placebo but not as effective as tetracycline. Erythromycin and clarithromycin[52] have also been shown to be useful alternatives to the tetracyclines.

Metronidazole was one of the first oral medications to have been used successfully for inflammatory rosacea.[65] The drug is now rarely used for rosacea because less toxic and more effective alternatives are available. One possible mode of action is via free radical scavenging activity.[66]

In an attempt at reducing the flushing and the degree of erythema seen in rosacea different blocking agents have been used including clonidine[67] and nadolol[68] but none of these has proved to be clinically useful.

Isotretinoin has been used for patients with severe persistent rosacea. The Cardiff group reported that oral isotretinoin did decrease the size of noses affected by rhinophyma[69] while the drug was administered but had no other therapeutic effect. Unfortunately the noses enlarged again after the isotretinoin was stopped. Others have found isotretinoin to be useful for some patients[70] – particularly for what has been termed rosacea fulminans. There are however, in the author's view, few instances when the drug is indicated for rosacea.

Oral terbinafine was found to help patients with papular rosacea in an open study, but as yet no confirmatory reports have appeared and no explanation has been advanced to account for any therapeutic activity.

Treatment of rhinophyma

The cosmetic results of treating rhinophyma surgically are really quite gratifying. There is little to choose between the various techniques which all involve some form of surgical sculpting of the deformed and hyperplastic tissue masses to a more normal nasal contour. Surgical paring and laser paring are probably the most popular methods – both giving excellent results cosmetically.

References

1. Wilkin J, Dahl M, Detmar M et al. Standard Grading System for Rosacea: report of the National Rosacea Society Expert Committee on the classification and staging of rosacea. J Am Acad Dermatol 2003; 46: 584–7.
2. Gupta AK, Chaudhry MM. Rosacea and its management – an overview. JEADV 2005; 19: 273–85.
3. Powell FC. Rosacea: Curse of the Celts. Poster presentation. Am Acad Dermatol 2001.
4. Long CC, Darke C, Marks R. Celtic ancestry, HLA phenotype and increased cancer. Br J Dermatol 1998; 138: 627–30.
5. Browning DJ, Rosenwasser G, Lugo M. Ocular rosacea in blacks. Am J Ophthalmol 1986; 10: 441–4.

6. Berg M, Liden S. An epidemiological study of rosacea. Acta Derm Venereol 1989; 69: 419–23.
7. Drolet B, Paller AS. Childhood rosacea. Paediatr Dermatol 1992; 9: 22–6.
8. Irvine C, Marks R. Prognosis and prognostic factors in rosacea. In: Marks R, Plewig G, eds. Acne and Related Disorders. Proceedings of an International Symposium. London: Martin Dunitz, 1989: 331–4.
9. Knight AK, Vickers CFH. A follow up of tetracycline treated rosacea. Br J Dermatol 1975; 93: 577–80.
10. Chaucer G. Prologue to the Canterbury Tales.
11. Shakespeare W. In Henry IV part I. Act 4. Scene 2.
12. Gajewska M. Rosacea of common male baldness. Br J Dermatol 1975; 93: 63–6.
13. Marks R, Wilson Jones E. Disseminated rosacea. Br J Dermatol 1969; 81: 16–28.
14. Rockl H, Germon J, Schropl F, Scherer M. Rosacea mit extrafacialer Lokalisation. Hautarzt 1969; 8: 348.
15. Helm KF, Menz J, Gibson LE, Dicken CH. A clinical and histopathologic study of granulomatous rosacea. J Am Acad Dermatol 1991; 253: 1038–43.
16. Borrie JP. The state of blood vessels of the face in rosacea. Br J Dermatol 1955; 67: 5.
17. Marks R, Beard RJ, Clark ML et al. Gastrointestinal observations in rosacea. Lancet 1967; 1: 739.
18. Bernardini FP, Kersten RC, Khouri LM. Chronic eyelid lymphoedema and acne rosacea. Report of two cases. Ophthalmology 2000; 107: 2220–3.
19. Gudmundsen KJ, O'Donnell BF, Powell FC. Schirmer testing for dry eyes in patients with rosacea. J Am Acad Dermatol 1992; 26: 211–14.
20. Motley RJ, Barton S, Marks R. The significance of telangiectasia in rosacea. In: Mars R, Pleura G, eds. Acne and Related Disorders. An International Symposium. London: Martin Dunitz, 1989: 339.
21. Marks R, Harcourt Webster N. Histopathology of rosacea. Arch Dermatol 1969; 100: 683–91.
22. Schmidt NF, Gans EH. Demodex and rosacea: the prevalence and numbers of Demodex mites in rosacea. Cos Dermatol 2004; 17: 497–502.
23. Skrlon J, Richter B, Basta-Juzbasic A et al. Demodicidosis and rosacea. Lancet 1991; 337: 734.
24. Ayres S Jr, Ayres S 3rd. Demodectic eruptions (demodicidosis) in the human. 30 years, experience with 2 commonly unrecognized entities: pityriasis folliculorum (Demodex) and acne rosacea (Demodex type). Arch Dermatol 1961; 83: 816–27.
25. Plesch E. A Rorschach study of rosacea and morbid blushing. Br J Med Psychol 1951; 24: 202–5.
26. Marks R. Concepts in the pathogenesis of rosacea. Br J Dermatol 1968; 80: 170–7.
27. Mackley CL. Body dysmorphic disorder. Dermatol Surg 2005; 31: 553–8.
28. Epstein N, Susnow D. Acne rosacea with particular reference to gastric secretion. Calif East Med 1930; 35: 118.
29. Søbye P. Aetiology and pathogenesis of rosacea. Acta Derm Venereol 1950; 30: 137.
30. Watson WC, Paton E, Murray D. Small bowel disease in rosacea. Lancet 1965; 2: 47.
31. Marks R, Beard RJ, Clark ML et al. Gastrointestinal observations in rosacea. Lancet 1967; 1: 739–43.
32. Sglachcic A. The link between Helicobacter pylori infection and rosacea. J EADV 2002; 16: 328–33.
33. Zentilin P, Brusati C, Puvari M et al. Prevalence of Helicobacter pylori infection in patients with rosacea. Gastroenterology 2000; 118 (Suppl 2).
34. Banford JTM, Tilden RM, Blankush RN et al. Effect of treatment of Helicobacter pylori infection on rosacea. Arch Dermatol 1999; 135: 659–63.
35. Erbagci Z, Özgöztasi O. The significance of Demodex follicularum density in rosacea. Int J Derm 1998; 37: 421–5.
36. Schmidt NF, Scott EH. Demodex and rosacea 1: the prevalence and numbers of Demodex mites in rosacea. Cos Dermatol 2004; 17: 497–502.
37. Ecker RI, Winkelmann RK. Demodex granuloma. Arch Dermatol 1979; 115: 343–4.

38. Lowe NJ, Henderson T, Millikan LE et al. Topical metronidazole for severe and recalcitrant rosacea. Cutis 1989; 43: 283–6.
39. Mond BE, Logan RA, Cook J et al. Topical metronidazole in the treatment of rosacea. J Dermatol Treat 1991; 2: 91–3.
40. Nielsen PG. A double blind study of 1% metronidazole cream versus systemic oxytetracycline therapy for rosacea. Br J Dermatol 1983; 109: 63–5.
41. Maddin S. A comparison of topical azelaic acid 20% cream in the treatment of patients with papulopustular rosacea. J Am Acad Dermatol 1999; 40: 961–5.
42. Carmichael AJ, Marks R, Graupe K et al. Topical azelaic acid in the treatment of rosacea. J Dermatol Treat 1993; 4: (Suppl 1) 519–22.
43. Maddin S. A comparison of topical azelaic acid 20% cream and topical metronidazole 0.75% cream in the treatment of patients with papulopustular rosacea. J Am Acad Dermatol 1999; 40: 961–5.
44. Elewski BE, Fleischer BE Jr, Pariser DM. A comparison of 15% azelaic acid gel and 0.75% metronidazole gel in the topical treatment of papulopustular rosacea. Arch Dermatol 2003; 139: 1444–50.
45. Thiboutot D, Thieroff-Ekerdt R, Graupe K. Efficacy and safety of azelaic acid (15%) gel as a new treatment for papulopustular rosacea. Results from the vehicle controlled randomized phase III studies. J Am Acad Dermatol 2003; 48: 836–45.
46. Sander DN, Miller R, Gratton D et al. The treatment of rosacea: the safety and efficacy of sodium sulfacetamide 10% and sulphur 5% lotion (Novacet) is demonstrated in a double blind study. J Dermatol Treat 1997; 1.
47. Torok HM, Webster G, Dunlap FE et al. Combination sodium sulfacetamide 10% and sulphur 5% with sunscreens versus metronidazole 0.75% cream for rosacea. Cutis 2005; 75: 357–63.
48. Kligman AM. Topical tretinoin for rosacea: a preliminary report. J Dermatol Treat 1993; 4: 41–73.
49. Vienne MP, Ochando N, Barrel MT. Retinaldehyde alleviates rosacea. Dermatology 1999; 199(Suppl 1): 53–6.
50. Altinyazar HC, Koca R, Tekin NS. Adapalene vs. metronidazole gel for the treatment of rosacea. Int J Dermatol 2005; 44: 252–5.
51. Wilkin J, De Witt. Treatment of rosacea. Topical clindamycin versus oral tetracycline. Int J Dermatol 1993; 32: 65–7.
52. McHugh RC, Rice A, Sangha ND, et al. A topical azithromycin preparation for the treatment of acne vulgaris and rosacea. J Dermatol Treat 2004; 15: 295–302.
53. Bamford JT, Elliott BA, Haller IV. Tacrolimus effect on rosacea. J Am Acad Dermatol 2004; 50: 107–8.
54. Crawford KM, Russ B, Bostram P. Pimecrolimus for treatment of acne rosacea. Skinmed 2005; 4: 147–50.
55. Draelos ZD, Fuller BB. Efficacy of 1% 4-ethoxybenzaldehyde in reducing facial erythema. J Dermatol Surg 2005; 31: 881–5.
56. Swenor ME. Is permethrin 5% cream effective for rosacea. J Fam Pract 2003; 52: 183–4.
57. Lowe NJ, Behr KL, Fitzpatrick R, Goldman M, Ruiz-Espanza J. Flash lamp pumped dye laser for rosacea – associated telangiectasia and erythema. J Dermatol Surg Oncol 1991; 17: 522–5.
58. Mark KA, Sparacio RM, Voigt A, Marenus K, Sarnoff DS. Objective and quantitative improvement of rosacea – associated erythema after intense pulsed light therapy. Dermatol Surg 2003; 29: 600–4.
59. Clarke SM, Lanigan SW, Marks R. Laser treatment of erythema and telangiectasia associated with rosacea. Lasers Med Sci 2002; 17: 26–33.
60. Spadin AN, Fleischmajer R. Tetracyclines: non-antibiotic properties and their clinical implications. J Am Acad Dermatol 2006; 54: 258–65.
61. Wojnarowska F, Kirtschig G, Khumalo N. Treatment of subepidermal immunobullous diseases. Clin Dermatol 2001; 19: 768–77.
62. Joshi RK, Atukorala DN, Abanmi A, al Khamis O, Haleem A. Successful treatment of Sweet's syndrome with doxycycline. Br J Dermatol 1993; 128: 584–6.
63. Marks R, Ellis J. Comparative effectiveness of tetracycline and ampicillin in rosacea. A controlled trial. Lancet 1971; 2: 1049–52.

64. Shapiro LE, Knowles SR, Shear NH. Comparative safety of tetracycline, minocycline and doxycyline. Arch Dermatol 1997; 133: 1224–30.
65. Pye RJ, Burton JL. Treatment of rosacea by metronidazole. Lancet 1976; 1: 1211–2.
66. Miyachi Y. Potential antioxidant mechanism of action for metronidazole: implications for rosacea management. Adv Ther 2001; 18: 237–43.
67. Wilkin JK. Effect of subdepressor clomidine on flushing reactions in rosacea. Arch Dermatol 1983; 119: 211–14.
68. Wilkin JK. Effect of nadolol on flushing reactions in rosacea. J Am Acad Dermatol 1989; 20: 202–5.
69. Irvine C, Kumar P, Marks R. Isotretinoin in the treatment of rosacea and rhinophyma. In: Marks, Plewig G, eds. Acne and Related Disorders. Proceedings of an International Symposium. London: Martin Dunitz, 1989: 301–5.
70. Mahrle G, Bauermeister-Jasso K, Endver K. Accutane therapy for acne and rosacea. Zeitschrift für Hautkrankheiten 1985; 60: 120–34.

3

Perioral dermatitis and miscellaneous inflammatory disorders of unknown origin

Definition

Perioral dermatitis (POD) may be defined as a not uncommon inflammatory disorder of facial skin of unknown cause in which small papules and pustules occur around the mouth and at the sides of the nose in young women predominantly.

Historical aspects

This disorder seems to have its roots in the second half of the 20th century as the first reports of a disease with its characteristic clinical features appeared in the 1950s. Unfortunately the various names used for the condition and the lack of clinical criteria for inclusion of patients make some aspects of the history somewhat uncertain.

It is generally accepted that the report of Frumess and Lewis in 1957[1] of what they termed 'light-sensitive seborrhoeid' was the first to describe the condition. A little later Mihan and Ayres[2] gave the condition the name 'perioral dermatitis', which has stuck, although other names were used such as 'rosacea-like dermatosis'.[3] Definitive descriptions were given by Cochran and Thomson[4] and Wilkinson et al.[5]

Clinical features

The disorder is surprisingly consistent in its clinical presentation. Characteristically the disorder first appears around the external nares and the superior end of the nasolabial folds or around the lip commissures (Figure 3.1). The eruption then spreads around the mouth leaving a clear and uninvolved zone immediately adjacent to the lips or sometimes separated from them by a thin clear zone. When severe and/or long-standing the condition travels up at the sides of the nose and may then even track laterally to involve the glabella. A curious variant has been described in which the disorder occurs predominantly around the eyes. This has come to be known as periocular perioral dermatitis[6] (Figure 3.2).

The basic lesions of POD are typically small papules (or micropapules) but

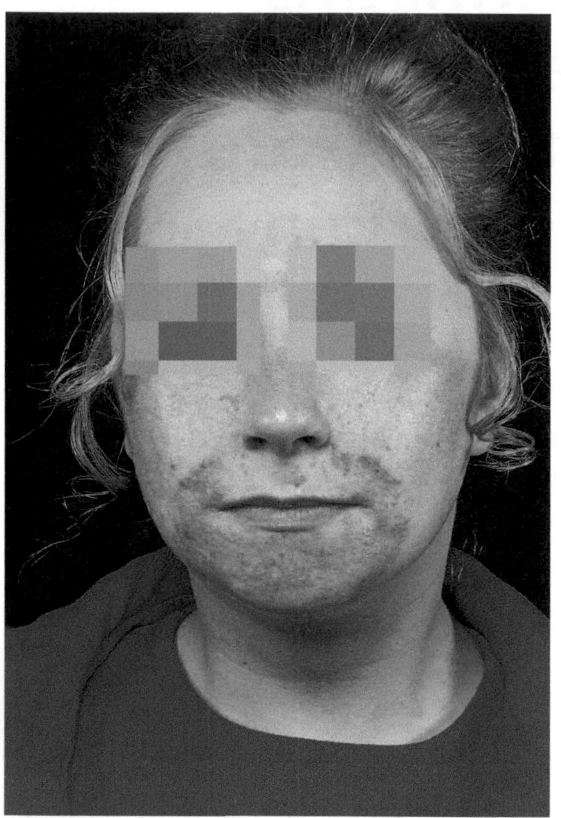

Figure 3.1

Typical distribution of perioral dermatitis with involvement of the skin around the mouth and the nasolabial grooves.

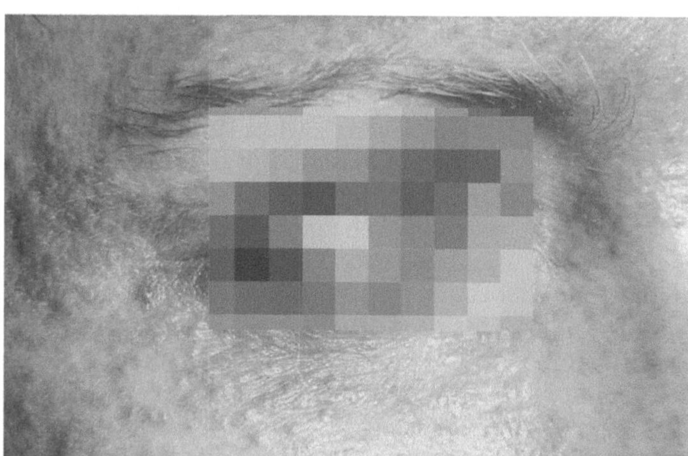

Figure 3.2

Perioral dermatitis like lesions around the eyes – so called 'periocular perioral dermatitis'.

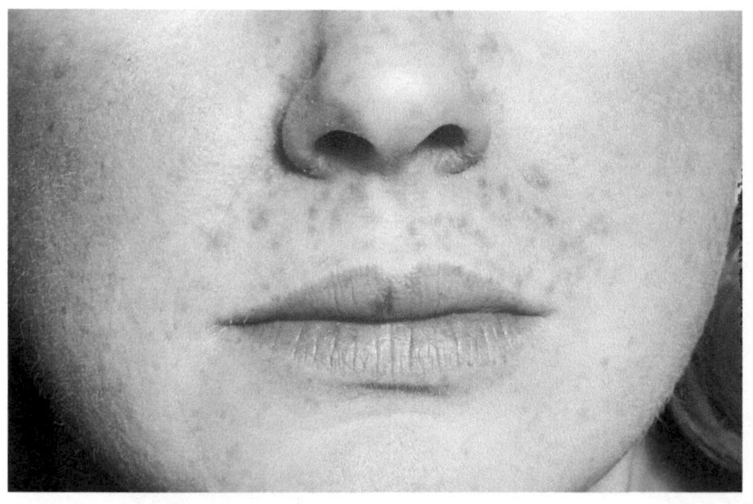

Figure 3.3

Early lesions of perioral dermatitis. The basic lesions are micropapules or papulopustules.

some of the lesions seem to be surmounted by tiny pustules as well as there being pustules occurring independently (Figure 3.3). Unlike rosacea there is no persistent erythema or telangiectasia although there may be a background faint pink flush on the affected skin and the papules themselves are a shade of red. As stated in the definition of the disease above, POD is predominantly a disease of young women (15–25 years). It is nonetheless also seen occasionally in young men – perhaps 5–10% occurring in men. Another variant that has been described is a granulomatous form occurring in children.[7] This disorder occurring in children of both sexes from 7 months to 13 years of age has similarities to rosacea and is marked histologically by a granulomatous infiltrate. Generally POD causes little in the way of symptoms apart from some mild soreness. The condition, nonetheless, causes considerable distress because of the prominent exposed position of the disorder on the face and the obvious cosmetic disturbance it causes.

Differential diagnosis

POD is easily differentiated from rosacea because the latter disorder occurs on facial convexities, is characterized by persistent erythema and telangiectasia with episodes of inflammation in which papules and pustules occur and is generally seen in mature adults of both sexes. POD is often confused with seborrheic dermatitis but this condition is scaly and itchy and may be exudative. The differentiation is made easier by the occurrence of dandruff as well as affected areas occurring elsewhere over the skin in seborrheic dermatitis particularly in the flexural areas.

The usual age group affected in POD may also lead the dermatologist to consider the possibility of acne. However, the different distribution of the rash over the face, the presence of lesions on the upper trunk in acne, the presence of comedones and seborrhea all serve to distinguish these two conditions.

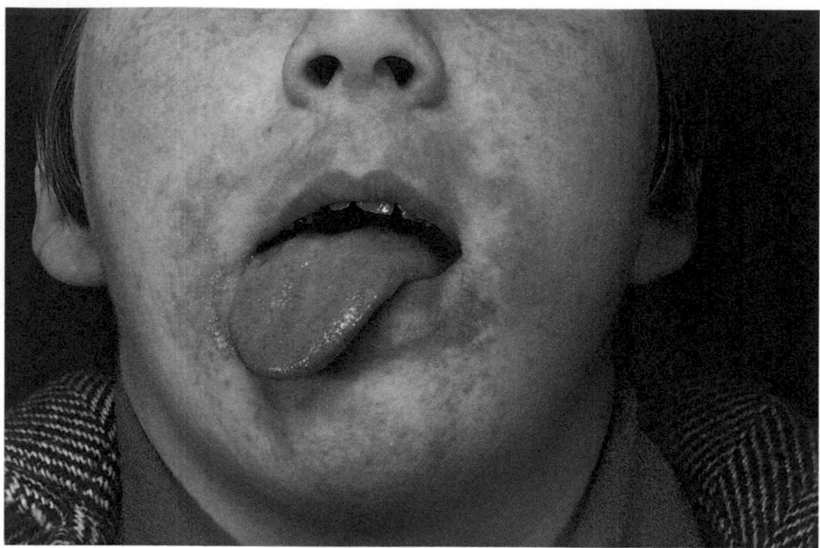

Figure 3.4

Lip licking cheilitis due to constant licking of the skin around the mouth.

The term dermatitis in POD is really a misnomer and it is important to differentiate forms of 'true' dermatitis from POD. One form of dermatitis that is quite distinctive and sometimes mistaken for POD is 'lip licking cheilitis' seen predominantly in the 7–15 years age group. In this disorder the rash is caused by the repeated licking of the skin around the mouth and is marked by skin scaling pink around the mouth and which is continuous with the vermilion (Figure 3.4). Allergic contact dermatitis to lip cosmetics can also result in a 'circumoral' dermatitis[8] but this is quite uncommon.

Course and prognosis

The condition usually arises spontaneously over the course of a week or two. In nearly every patient there is a striking dependency on topical corticosteroids. A frequently heard story is that the patient presents with the earliest signs of the rash and is given a potent or moderately potent topical corticosteroid. The condition then shows some improvement but when an attempt is made to stop treatment the condition dramatically worsens after a few days. This happens every time they try to leave off the steroid preparation. In fact the condition tends to be doggedly persistent and there does not seem to be any tendency to spontaneous remission. Luckily the correct treatment with antibiotics cures the condition (see below).

Epidemiology

The condition is mainly a disease of women aged 15–25 but occasionally it is

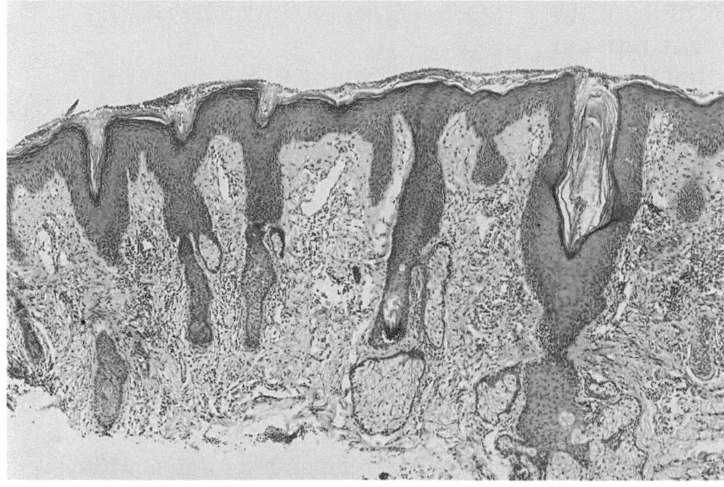

Figure 3.5

Photomicrograph of section from biopsy of perioral dermatitis. There is some inflammatory cell infiltrate in the dermis and minimal spongiotic change in the follicular epithelium.

seen in children.[9,10] There are no validated data on the frequency of the disease and it may well be that the incidence varies in different countries. In the UK it seemed at one time to be a very common disorder in routine dermatological practice but then in the 1980s is seemed to vanish and become quite uncommon but it showed a resurgence in the 1990s. The same sequence does not seem to have been the case in the USA and some other countries from which reports of studies and case reports have continued to appear[11,12] in a steady stream.

Pathology

There have been few studies of the microscopic pathology of POD presumably because of the reluctance of clinicians to biopsy the facial skin of young women. However, 3 or even 4 mm diameter punch biopsy rarely produces a significant scar in inflamed facial skin if no sutures are inserted. Our study of 26 patients demonstrated the presence of eczematous changes predominantly, with most of the spongiotic change being focused on the external root sheaths of the follicles (Figure 3.5). In this investigation there did not appear to be any similarity to the pathological changes noted in rosacea.[13] Ramelet[14] did not share this view and stated that in his series of 30 cases the changes were most like those of rosacea. In one series of POD in children a granulomatous reaction was a consistent finding and this often appeared to emanate from follicular rupture.

The cause(s) of POD

As yet no convincing explanation to account for the cause of this disease has emerged. The striking predominance in women, the relationship with topical corticosteroid treatment and the curious sudden appearance of the disorder in the 1950s/60s have been difficult to fit together into any coherent rational hypothesis. The early view that it was in some way light-induced has not been sustained and most writers on the topic have focused on either an infective cause or the result of some form of topical application. Both *Candida* yeasts and fusiform bacteria have been considered as possible etiological agents but evidence in support has not been forthcoming.[15,16] The demodex mite has also been accused of causing the eruption[17] but although demodex may cause some facial rashes there is no evidence of its involvement in POD. Cosmetics have been often considered as causative agents of the condition. If this is the case then physical occlusion or some form of irritation (? follicular irritation) may be responsible. Certainly allergic contact dermatitis does not seem a likely candidate as patch tests to various cosmetic agents have been consistently negative.[18] Contact with bristly male chin beard stubble has been discussed as a cause but has been hotly denied as a possibility by some patients. Fluoride-containing toothpaste[19,20] and/or fluoridation of water supplies has been blamed but has received no further support.

Most attention has been given to potent topical corticosteroids, particularly fluorinated topical corticosteroids as causative agents.[21,22] It is certainly the case that many subjects develop a strange dependency on the use of these steroid creams and flare when they stop using them but this is a long way from saying that they actually cause the disorder. It has to be borne in mind that a small number of patients vigorously deny ever having used topical corticosteroids.

Management of patients with POD

Most patients are anxious and depressed by the time they reach the dermatologist because of the succession of ineffective treatments they have had. Strong reassurance concerning the eventual successful outcome is needed. Right at the start of treatment all topical corticosteroids should be stopped and the patient should be warned that a flare of the rash will almost certainly develop within a few days, but will only last for a few days. Some have suggested that a weak corticosteroid such as hydrocortisone should be given during this period, but this does not stop the flare or alleviate the symptoms in most patients. It is probably better to experience the flare 'cold turkey' using just an emollient and continuing to take one of the oral tetracyclines (see below).

Most patients respond to oral tetracycline, either tetracycline itself or one of the more recent analogs such as minocycline, doxycyline or lymecycline. These drugs should be given in full dosage until the patient starts to respond – usually a 3 or 4 week period – and then reduced to half dosage until the rash has completely resolved. Usually treatment can be stopped after 8–10 weeks. Recurrences are very uncommon and luckily there are no sequelae. The mode of action of the tetracyclines does not appear to be purely antimicrobial and is yet another of the mysteries associated with POD. Other oral antibiotics have been used such as erythromycin and have been claimed as successful. Topical metronidazole,[23] topical erythromycin and topical tetracycline[24] have all been used, but it is rare that such therapies are required.

Acne agminata (syn. lupus miliaris disseminatus faciei; acnitis)

Definition

Acne agminata may be defined as a very uncommon inflammatory disorder of unknown cause affecting skin of the face and upper trunk characterized by the appearance of persistent dark red to brown acneiform papules.

Clinical features

Non-tender brownish red papules develop over one to several weeks anywhere over the face or upper trunk (Figure 3.6). There is no tendency to form pustules, they arise on normal-appearing skin without any hint of erythema or telangiectasia. They have an 'indolent' appearance and behave as suggested by their appearance. They stubbornly persist for many months or even years and then resolve without any warning. In one series most lesions disappeared within 2–4 years.[25] When they do depart they leave a reminder of their presence in the shape of a pock-like scar. No concomitant clinical abnormalities have been described.

In the differential diagnosis the most important differentials are acne and rosacea, but the presence of the papules without accompanying abnormalities, the story of persistence of the papules and their characteristic appearance should lead to the correct diagnosis.

Pathology

The changes are essentially those of a dermal granuloma. There are large foci of mononuclear cells towards the center of which are larger macrophage-type cells, epithelioid cells and scattered giant cells. In addition there is central caseation necrosis – just as is seen in lupus vulgaris (Figure 3.7). No foreign material or remnants of microbes can be detected – although it should be noted that the PCR technique has been reported to detect mycobacterial traces in the granulomata.

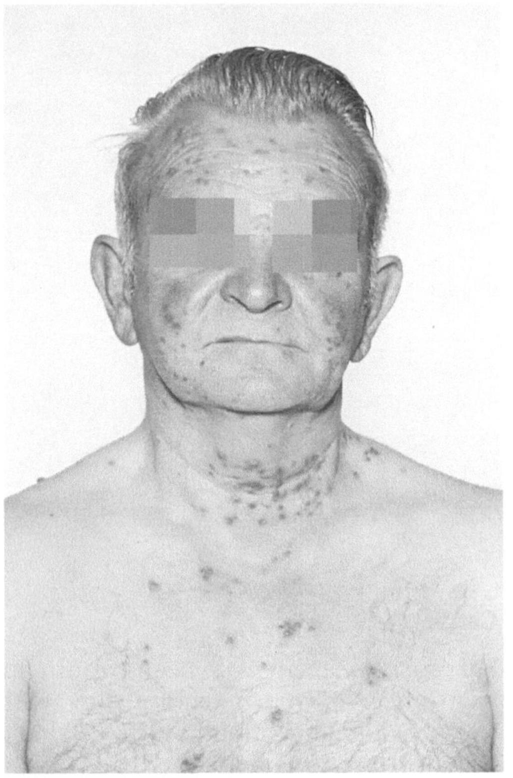

Figure 3.6

Acne agminata. This patient has persistent inflammatory papules on his upper chest, neck and cheek.

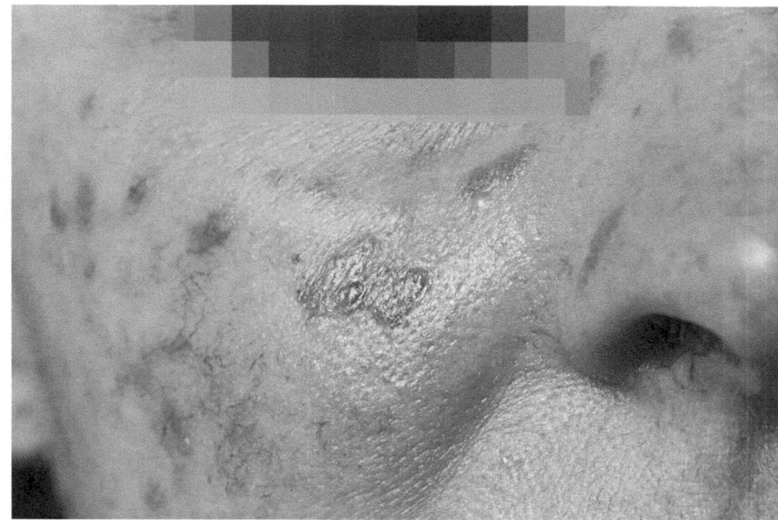

Figure 3.7

Brown-red plaque of granuloma faciale.

Cause

No causative agency has been confirmed. As noted above a relationship with mycobacterial infection has been claimed but no other evidence has been forthcoming.

Management

Treatments for acne, rosacea, perioral dermatitis, lupus vulgaris and autoimmune disorders appear to have little or no effect.[25] Treatment with dapsone, corticosteroids and thalidomide are likewise disappointingly ineffectual. Treatment with 'biologics' has not been reported at the time of writing.

Granuloma faciale

This is a curious and quite rare condition in which red-brown or occasionally violaceous plaques or nodules develop over the face. In most instances solitary lesions are found but occasionally multiple lesions develop. The condition predominates in adult males[26] mostly appearing on the forehead or cheeks. Rarely extrafacial lesions occur.[27] The condition persists for very long periods and is subject to remission and relapse. The name is somewhat inappropriate as histologically there is little evidence of granulomatous inflammation. In a recent analysis[26] of biopsies from 66 cases it was found that lymphocytes were the most frequent inflammatory cells present, followed by neutrophils and plasma cells. Eosinophils were present in 57% biopsies and leukocytoclasis was found in some 66%. Other notable features were a clear zone sub-epidermally (Grenz zone) and obvious damage to capillary endothelium with the inflammation often being predominantly perivascular. This picture is 'vasculitic' and more reminiscent of erythema elevatum diutinum than a granuloma. Interestingly granuloma faciale has been noted to occur in association with an unusual fibrotic condition affecting the mucosa of the upper respiratory tract known as eosinophilic angiocentric fibrosis.[28] Histologically, this latter disorder is identical to granuloma faciale.

Treatment with the pulsed dye laser was successful in two of four patients[29] but in all patients treated by cryotherapy.[30]

Cheilitis granulomatosa (syn Melkersson–Rosenthal syndrome)

This is a rare disorder of unknown origin characterized by persistent swelling of a lip, facial nerve palsy and stable fissured tongue (lingua plicata). Extensive investigation usually fails to reveal a cause. The condition is usually resistant to all forms of treatment though in one report a patient appeared to respond to intralesional injections with triamcinolone.

References

1. Frumess GM, Lewis HM. Light-sensitive seborrheid. AMA Arch Dermatol 1957; 75: 245–8.
2. Mihan R, Ayres S. Perioral dermatitis. Arch Dermatol 1964; 89: 803–5.
3. Editorial. Rosacea like dermatitis. BMJ 1969; 3: 545.
4. Cochran REI, Thomson J. Perioral dermatitis. J Clin Exper Dermatol 1979; 4: 75.
5. Wilkinson DS, Kirton V, Wilkinson JD. Perioral dermatitis. Br J Dermatol 1979; 101: 245.
6. Fisher AA. Perioocular dermatitis akin to the perioral variety. J Am Acad Dermatol 1986; 15: 642–4.
7. Tarm K, Creel NB, Kruvda SJ, Turiansky GW. Granulomatous periorificial dermatitis. Cutis 2004; 73: 399–402.
8. Bandl BJ. Perioral dermatitis: etiology and treatment. Cutis 1976; 17: 903–8.
9. Manders M, Lucky AW. Perioral dermatitis in childhood. J Am Acad Dermatol 1992; 27: 688.
10. Laude TA, Salvemini JN. Perioral dermatitis in children. Semin Cutan Med Surg 1999; 18: 206–9.
11. Hafeez ZH. Perioral dermatitis: an update. Int J Dermatol 2003; 42: 514–17.
12. Weber K, Thurmayr R. Critical appraisal of reports on the treatment of perioral dermatitis. Dermatology 2005; 210: 300–7.
13. Marks R, Black MM. Perioral dermatitis: a histopathological study of 26 cases. Br J Dermatol 1971; 84: 242.
14. Ramelet AA, Delacretax J. Etude histopathologique de la dermatite périorale. Dermatologica 1981; 163: 361–9.
15. Bradford LG, Montes LF. Perioral dermatitis and Candida albicans. Arch Dermatol 1972; 105: 892.
16. Buck A, Kalkoff AW. Zur Nachweis von Fusobakterien aus Effloreszenzen der peroralen dermatitis. Haugarzt 1971; 22: 433.
17. Bendl BJ. Perioral dermatitis: etiology and treatment. Cutis 1976; 17: 903.
18. Kaufman WH. Facial dermatitis of unknown cause. J Am Acad Dermatol 1965; 192: 252.
19. Epstein E. Fluoride toothpastes as a cause of acne-like eruptions. Arch Dermatol 1976; 112: 1033.
20. Saunders MA. Fluoride toothpastes: a cause of acne-like eruptions. Arch Dermatol 1975; 111: 793.
21. Cotterill JA. Perioral dermatitis. Br J Dermatol 1979; 101: 259–62.
22. Wilkinson DS, Kirton V, Wilkinson JD. Perioral dermatitis: a 12 year review. Br J Dermatol 1979; 101: 245–57.
23. Miller SR, Shalita AR. Topical metronidazole gel for the treatment of perioral dermatitis in children. J Am Acad Dermatol 1994; 31: 847.
24. Wilson RG. Topical tetracycline in the treatment of perioral dermatitis. Arch Dermatol 1979; 115: 637.
25. Borhan R, Vignon Pennamen MD, Morel P. Lupus miliaris disseminatus faciei: (6 cases). Ann Dermatol Venereol 2005; 132: 526–30.

26. Ortonne N, Weschler J, Bagot M. Granuloma faciale. A clinicopathologic study of 66 patients. J Am Acad Dermatol 2005; 53: 1002–9.
27. Oleun MR, Bauman L, Minor D. Granuloma faciale with lesions on the face and hand. Arch Dermatol 1965; 92: 78–80.
28. Navayan J, Douglas-Jones AG. Eosinophilic angiocentric fibrosis and granuloma faciale: analysis of cellular infiltrate and review of literature. Ann Otol Rhinol Laryngol 2005; 114: 35.
29. Cheung ST, Lanigan SW. Granuloma faciale treated with the pulsed-dye laser: a case series. Clin Exp Dermatol 2005; 30: 373–5.
30. Panagiotopoulos V, Anyfantakis E, Rallis V et al. Assessment of the efficacy of cryosurgery in the treatment of granuloma faciale. Br J Dermatol 2006; 154: 357–60.

Acne vulgaris

The term acne should be restricted to the disorder often known as acne vulgaris and not used for other papular disorders of facial skin such as rosacea (see pages 5). It may be defined as a common disorder of hair-bearing skin in which the follicular canal tends to become blocked by keratinous debris (comedones) and then becomes inflamed. Acne vulgaris is probably the commonest of all skin disorders and has an immense range of clinical expression and subtypes. Not unexpectedly ideas concerning its pathogenesis and the range of treatments and management strategies available are also extensive. Clearly I will only be able to deal with the 'headlines' of the topic and suggest that the reader consult some of the more comprehensive texts when fuller knowledge is required.[1,2]

Acne – who does it affect?

Acne can affect all humans with hair follicles. It is no respecter of ethnic type, geographical origin, socioeconomic class, gender, or even age. Accurate surveys do not appear to have been reported and so it is not possible to contrast the comparative frequency or severity of disease in different groups. All that can be done is to provide our professional experience and anecdotal views.

The disease first starts to make an impact at the time of puberty – 12–14 years of age. It then continues to cause problems, in many subjects, right up to the early years of the third decade. But these are 'broad brush strokes' and we should not be surprised at individuals who continue to develop lesions throughout their middle years or others who have one short sharp attack in the early teenage years and then just do not seem to be troubled again. It has been said that everyone experiences some acne at some time and the sometimes used term 'physiological acne' does indeed imply that in a mild form it is a normal occurrence. Acne can occur in infancy and may also appear in old age for the first time – these will be discussed a little later in this chapter.

The clinical signs of acne

Non-inflamed lesions

Important clinical signs of acne are excess greasiness of the skin – often known as seborrhea – and the presence of blackheads (comedones). Measurements made on the rate of sebum secretion per unit area of skin using either the older cigarette paper collection technique or a more modern optical method (e.g. sebumeter[3]) confirm that patients with clinical acne secrete sebum at a faster rate than do non-acne controls.[4] It is also the case that there is a linear relationship between the rate of secretion and the severity of the acne.[5] The greasy skin gives a distinctive sheen to the skin surface (Figure 4.1). It is uncommonly itself the cause of complaints but is nonetheless of cosmetic concern in many patients and an annoying inconvenience.

Comedones are either of the open or closed varieties. It is the former that are the most noticeable with their blackened superficial tips (Figure 4.2). They are commonly seen over the sides of the nose or over the forehead. It is not the open comedone that seems to be the starting point of the troublesome inflammatory lesions but the so-called closed comedones. These are not easily visible but are presumably found everywhere that inflammatory lesions occur.

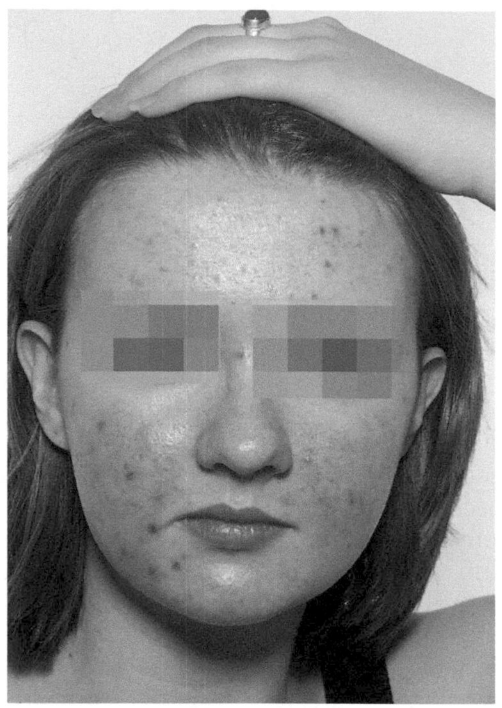

Figure 4.1

This young woman has a minor degree of acne but obvious seborrhea with 'shiny greasy skin'.

Inflammatory lesions

These are what most patients recognize as acne. Inflamed lesions include papules, pustules, papulopustules, nodules and cysts. Such lesions are often painful and tender and may be surrounded by a pink/red halo. They are irregular in shape

Figure 4.2

The 'blackheads' of open comedones are easily seen in this close-up photograph alongside resolving papules and scars.

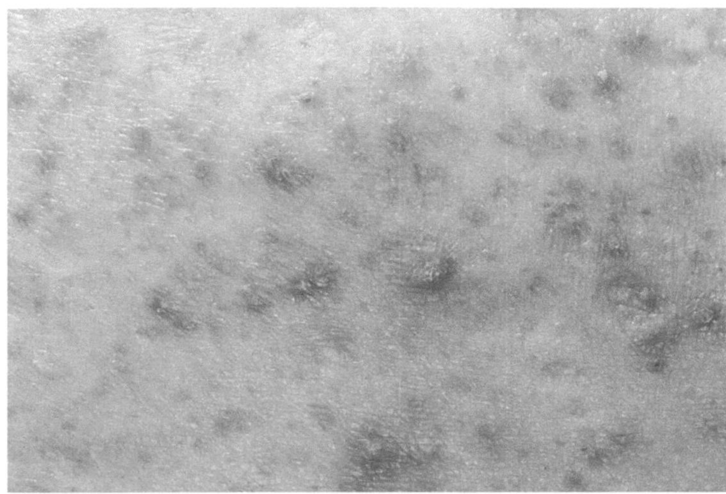

Figure 4.3

There are many papules of different shapes and sizes in this area of skin.

and are frequently at different stages of development even in the same anatomical field (Figure 4.3). Some papules develop whitish or yellowish white tips – as papulopustules. These latter do not stay very long as their owners tend to squeeze them or 'pop' them when performing their toilet. Some papules develop into stubborn deeply set papules or nodules which seem to defy most forms of treatment and are one of major cosmetic concern to their owners.

In patients with severe acne the inflamed lesions progress and coalesce so that a deep cystic lesion is formed. Purists in the dermatopathology world remind us that the term cyst for these lesions is inappropriate as there is no epithelial cyst lining in acne cysts. They are really just cold abscesses containing viscous or semisolid necrotic tissue and myriads of inflammatory cells – mostly polymorphs. Clinically these lesions are irregular in shape and vary in size from 0.5–3.0 cm in diameter and in color from skin color to all shades of red (Figures 4.4a and 4.4b). When acutely inflamed they are painful and tender and when more than one is present, as is often the case, they make their owner feel wretched.

Sequelae

The inflammatory lesions of acne are destructive and result in scars of which there are several types. The most deforming are keloid scars, which are luckily the least common. *Keloid scars* tend to occur on the front of the chest and over the shoulder and are more common in men than in women in the 15–20-year old age group (Figure 4.5). Keloid scars seem to form more readily in patients of African ancestry. They are unpredictable in that the size and degree of inflammation of the initial lesion bear little relationship to the ultimate size of the keloid, which is, anyway, by definition larger than the initiating damaging stimulus. Keloid scars may be itchy but the main disability from them is the disfigurement that they cause.

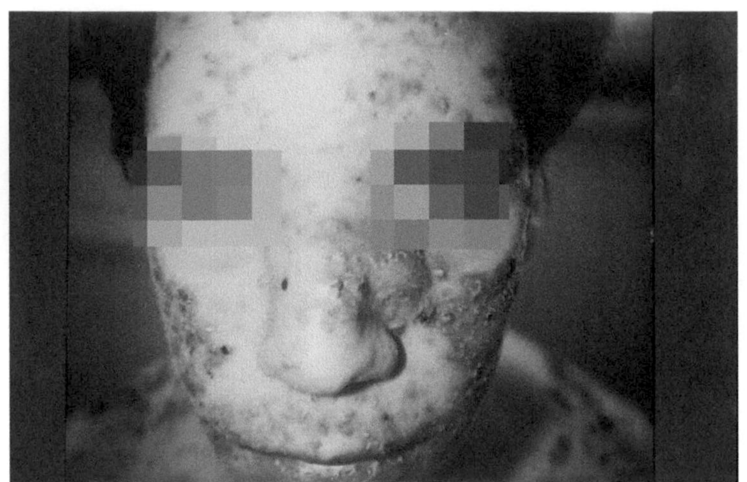

Figure 4.4a

This young man with severe acne has developed a cystic lesion at the side of the nose.

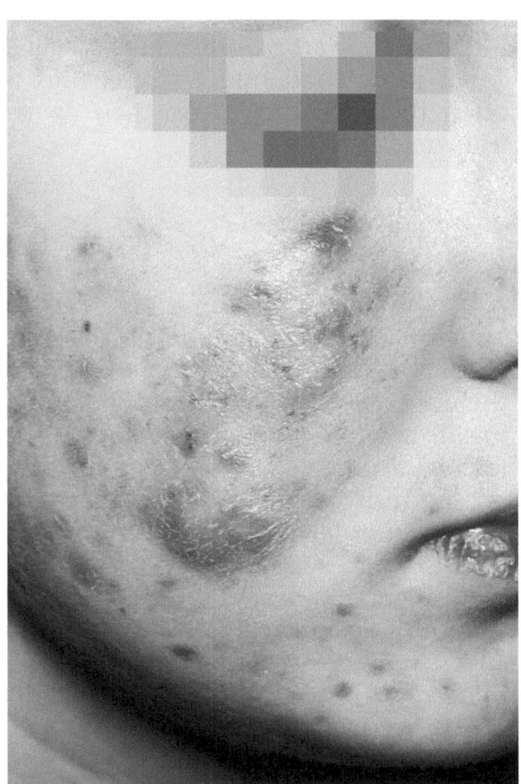

Figure 4.4b

Acne cyst on cheek.

Hypertrophic scars are less uncommon than keloids and are particularly frequently seen after severe acne over the shoulders, back and chest. They are pinkish and smooth with rounded contours (Figure 4.6). Sometimes there is linear 'bridging' nearby areas of severe inflammation. Unlike keloids they tend to flatten and become less prominent with time.

Pits look like their name suggests and are deep pits set in the skin surface. They are very common and although unloved by their owners are generally by themselves not a major cause of cosmetic discomfort.

Icepick scars are small triangular depressed areas which like pitted scars tend to become less prominent with time.

Which sites are involved?

All hair-bearing sites can be affected but areas with terminal hair are not usually involved with ordinary acne. The face,

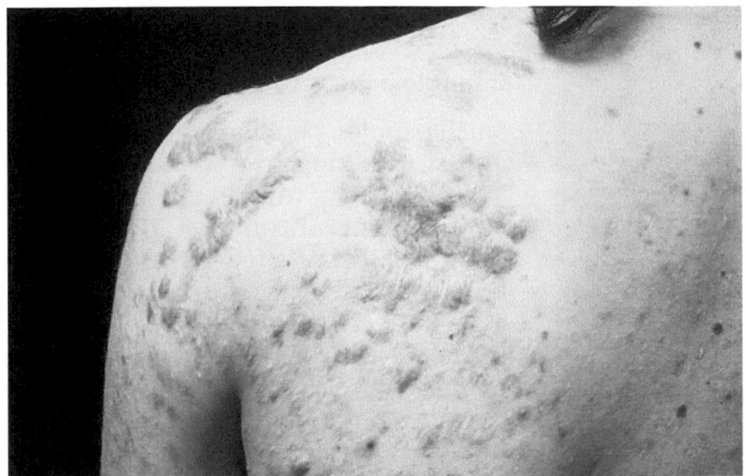

Figure 4.5

Keloid scars affecting the shoulder.

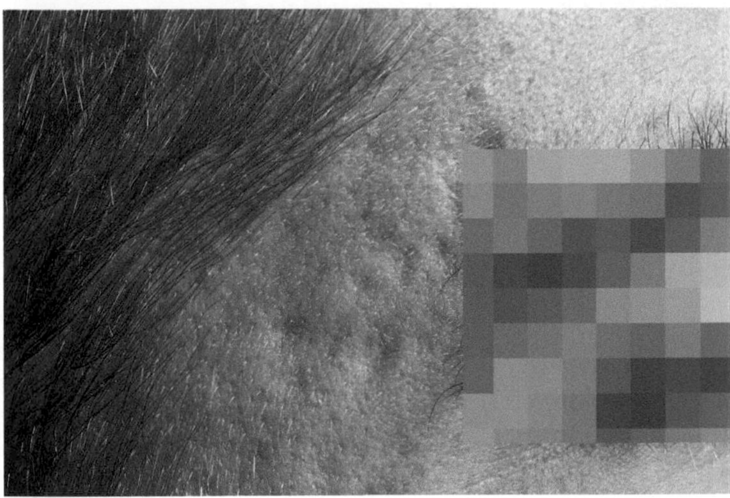

Figure 4.6

Shallow pock scars from acne.

shoulders, back of neck, upper back and front of chest are most often affected but the upper arms, the buttocks and thighs may all develop lesions in severely affected patients (Figure 4.7).

The majority of patients have at least two or three sites affected – a common pattern being the face and the upper back or the face, back and front of chest. On the face, the forehead, the jaw line, the sides of the neck and the cheeks are the most often affected.

Course of disease

In the large majority of patients the disease is trivial and these individuals

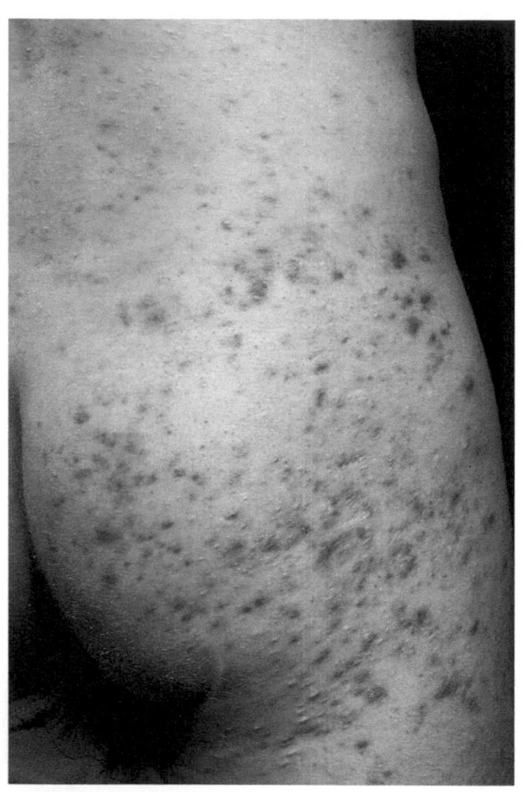

Figure 4.7

Acne involving buttock and thigh.

never reach a dermatologist. Many do not seek any form of medical advice at all but make do by using topical remedies from the supermarket or the pharmacy or even by the more convenient method of ignoring the problem. Acne is commonplace (some would say universal) around puberty, 12–14, but is usually trivial not requiring much more than reassurance. In most of those in whom acne lesions spread and continue to appear the disorder continues remittently for 2–4 years. In a few, however, the disease continues into the third and fourth decades and even longer.

Clinical variants

Infantile acne

Small papules, papulopustules and comedones appearing over the cheeks, nose and forehead of infants, a few months of age, are not uncommon (Figure 4.8). They usually last a few weeks or months but some have suggested that infantile acne indicates the development of acne in later years. The lesions are restricted to the face, are usually few in number and are for the most part superficial. It is rare that cysts develop (Figure 4.9).

Acne in mature age groups[6]

One sort of 'mature' acne is due to the persistence of acne through the third decade right up to mid-life and even beyond. Apart from its recalcitrant nature there is nothing special about this sort of acne from the clinical point of view. Another variety is seen in women in the third, fourth and fifth decades. It is curious in that there seems to be a predilection for involvement of the skin of the chin and a characteristic aggravation premenstrually. A third type of acne affecting mature age groups is a quite severe papular or cystic acne suddenly developing in subjects (usually men) in the fifth to eighth decades. This is mainly a disorder of truncal skin in men (Figure 4.9a). This sometimes appears to have been precipitated by a systemic disorder but in most instances no special precipitant can be identified.

Acne fulminans

This condition is of acute onset and extreme severity. It develops quite abruptly

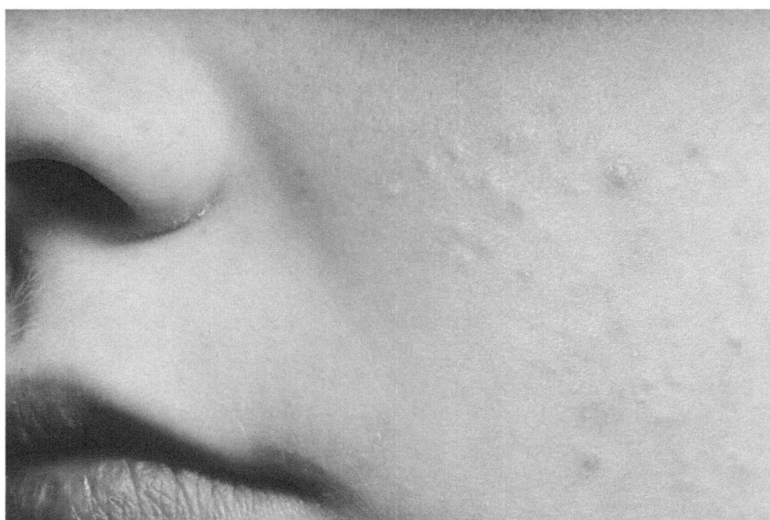

Figure 4.8

Infantile acne.

in the course of moderately severe unremarkable acne. Numerous large painful papules, nodules and cysts (Figures 4.10 and 4.10a) develop within the course of a few days accompanied by malaise, fever and a marked polymorphonuclear leukocytosis – sometimes of leukemoid proportions. In addition some patients suffer from a painful arthropathy of large and medium-sized joints and in a few splenomegaly develops. X-rays of the long bones sometimes reveal what appear to be punched-out holes. Their significance is not clear. What causes this severe systemic upset is unknown, but it does appear to have been precipitated by treatment with isotretinoin in a few instances.

Patients with acne fulminans require treatment with systemic antibiotics (such as doxycycline), systemic steroids, dapsone and topical medications at various times. The condition usually resolves after a few weeks or months.

Acne necrotica

This is usually divided into acne necrotica varioliformis and acne necrotica miliaris. The first form is characterized, as its name suggests, by the leaving of large varioliform scars, while the second is so named because there are many similar but much smaller lesions. Acne necrotica is quite uncommon, the miliaris type being the more frequent. Clinically, lesions are conical brown/red papules which may be topped by a blackish crust. They occur over the forehead, scalp and temple. The cause is unknown and the relationship to ordinary acne is uncertain. There is no special form of treatment but luckily the condition usually remits after some months.

Cosmetic acne

This condition became prominent some 30–40 years ago, but is now relatively uncommon. This is presumably because

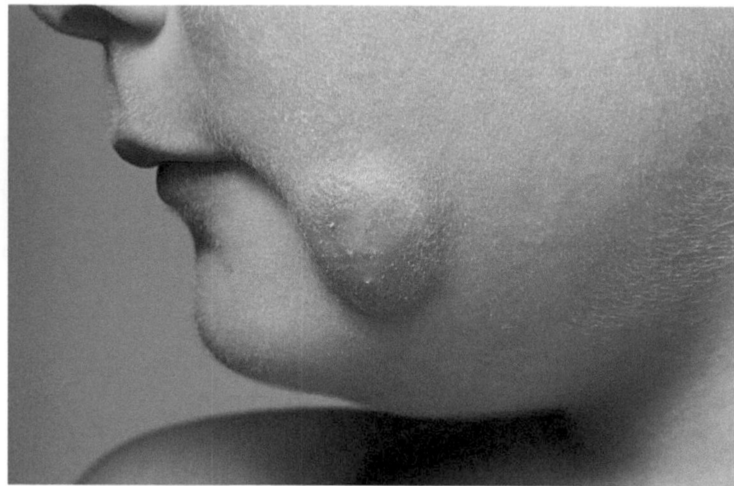

Figure 4.9

Cystic lesion due to infantile acne.

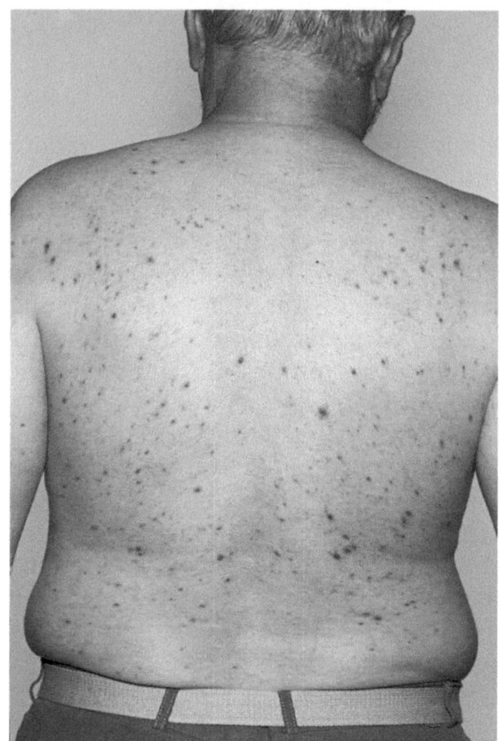

Figure 4.9a

Acne on back of 62-year-old man.

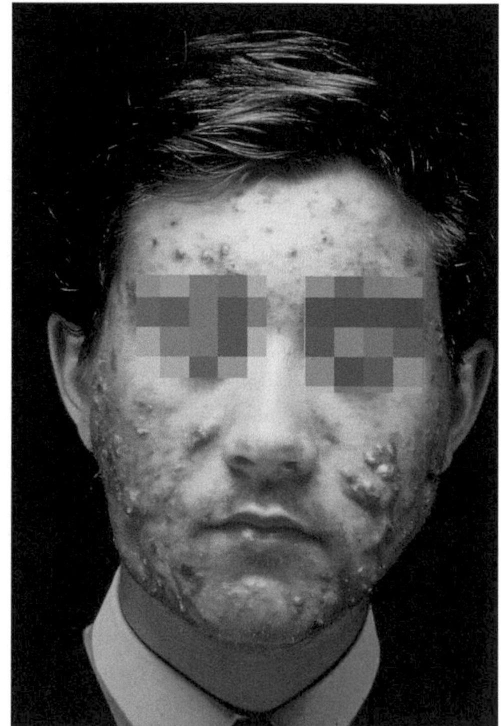

Figure 4.10

Acne fulminans.

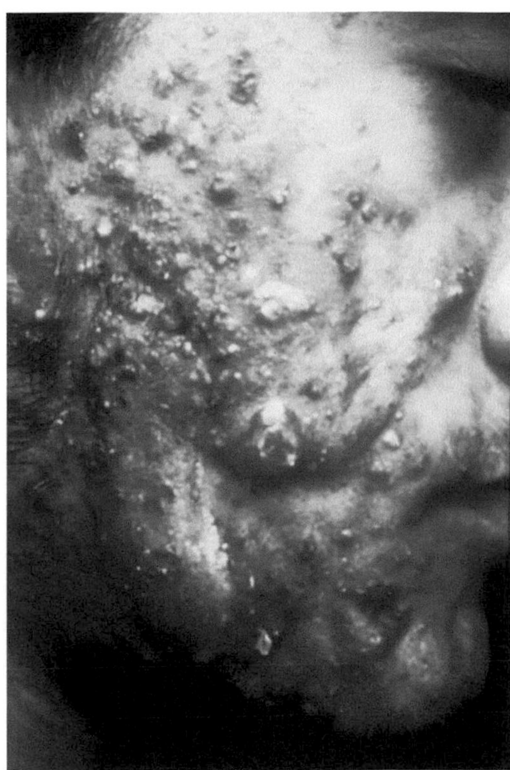

Figure 4.10a

Acne fulminans.

many of the causative agents in cosmetics that were responsible (comedogens or acneigens) have been replaced by blameless substances. The lesions of cosmetic acne usually affect one or two areas uniformly and consist of comedones, micropapules and papulopustular lesions. Cosmetics containing cocoa butter and derivatives, isopropyl myristate, tar products and paraffin hydrocarbons have been the main culprits, but less commonly, other agents can be responsible. Once the condition is identified and the offending cosmetic is stopped the lesions will remit – encouraged by a topical retinoid (see later). Cosmetics are still tested for their comedogenic potential by applying them to rabbit ears over some weeks and then examining the ears histologically.[7] This test has been superseded by a similar test in man[8] which unfortunately is not as sensitive.

Acne excoriée des jeunes filles

Why this extremely common type of acne should have a French name is not clear. It certainly is seen in acne sufferers of both sexes, all nationalities and ethnic types. It is however, as the name implies, mostly a problem of young female acne sufferers. Most patients with facial acne squeeze, pick or scratch their lesions – often in front of a mirror, in the vain attempt at trying to rid themselves of the tiresome and appearance-threatening spots. In some individuals the manual interference seems to become a major obsession and no spot is left unpicked (Figure 4.11). Advice and even stern instruction seems to have little effect – which is sad because the excoriated lesions stay longer and are more likely to lead to scarring. There are a few patients with very little real acne to see – only excoriations and inflamed spots around the scratches. These latter complain bitterly about their 'acne' and how resistant it is to treatment. Whether or not they start off by having a few acne spots is not certain. Acne excorieé, when severe, should be considered part of the dysmorphophobia syndrome.[9]

Androgen-induced acne

Typical acne lesions often develop during treatment with androgens given for whatever reason. Although anabolic

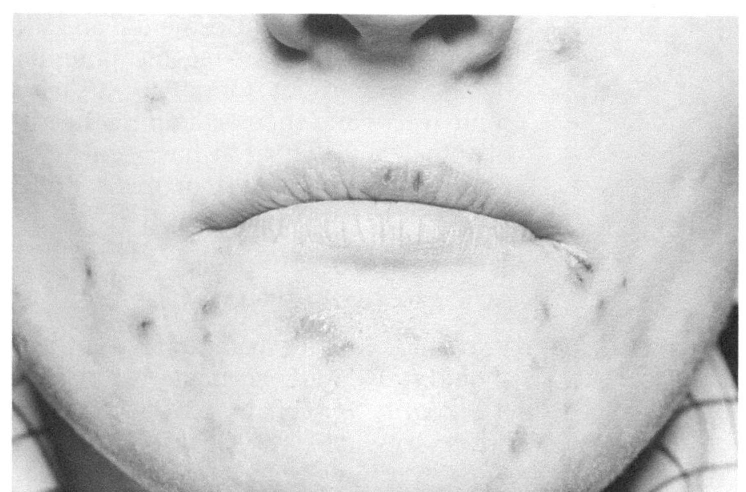

Figure 4.11

Acne excoriée – there are many small excoriated papules on the chin and at the sides of the mouth.

steroids have supposedly little in the way of masculinizing effects they are certainly capable of causing quite severe acne. This is sometimes a problem in 'body-builders' and it is always worthwhile asking young men with acne if they have been taking 'anything' by mouth to improve their muscles.

Acne is also part of the clinical picture of virilization seen in arrhenoblastoma (an ovarian androgen-producing tumor), an adrenocortical tumor or adrenocortical hyperplasia. There is also excess androgen production in the polycystic ovary disease (PCOS) and acne is also a problem in this group of young women.[10] The condition should be suspected in overweight young women with acne, hirsutism and menstrual irregulaties. It is surprisingly common, occurring in 3–5% of the female population.[11] Diagnosis of PCOS is confirmed by the blood levels of androgenic steroids and sex hormone-binding globulin while pelvic ultrasound will reveal the ovarian cysts.

Steroid-induced acne

Acne lesions frequently develop as a sign of hypercortisonism whether spontaneous as in Cushing's syndrome or iatrogenic due to treatment with glucocorticoids. The acne lesions are distinctive in that they tend to be small and are all at the same stage of development at a particular site. Comedones and cysts are not seen in 'steroid acne'. The lesions can occur anywhere but are commonly truncal.

Drug-induced acne

It is often stated that a drug such as isoniazid is capable of causing an acneiform eruption. If this is the case it must be extremely uncommon and the evidence incriminating non-hormonal drugs as a cause of acne is extremely slim.

Comedone nevus (see also Chapter 10)

This congenital disorder is characterized by the presence of patches of skin of various sizes and shapes at one or several sites containing large numbers of comedones (Figure 4.12). The only reason for including this odd nevoid disorder here is that the comedones sometimes give rise to inflammatory papules and this may help in the understanding of ordinary acne.

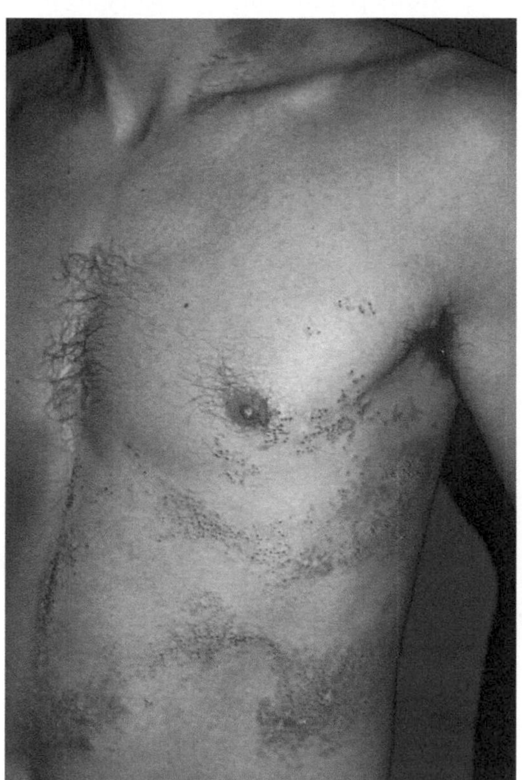

Figure 4.12

Comedone nevus. There are myriads of comedones in curving bands around the trunk.

Occupational acne

Repeated exposure to oils and greases causes the formation of comedones and sometimes inflamed papular lesions on the soiled skin. It seems that the oils have a particular irritant effect on the mouths of hair follicles. Mechanics and machine operators seem particularly at risk. Forearms and the fronts of thighs are particularly vulnerable. Contact with oil-soaked clothing seems to be a particular risk factor.

Chloracne is a persistent and serious variety of occupational acne due to systemic exposure to extraordinarily small amounts of the extremely potent group of substances known as dioxin which are by-products of a number of industrial chemical processes. Dioxin has caused major problems in a number of chemical plant disasters including that at Serveso in Italy and is notorious for being the agent used to poison a Ukrainian presidential candidate in recent years.[12] A major clinical manifestation of this poisoning is the appearance of numerous large acne-type cysts. The condition is terribly deforming, very persistent and unfortunately quite resistant to treatment.

Pathology

Acne is essentially a folliculitis which does not stay confined to the follicle. The initial lesion morphologically is the comedone (or blackhead). This black-tipped compaction of horny debris, inspissated sebum and the remains of follicular microflora has long been the subject of many colorful myths. It is the starting point of all the other lesions of acne.

It is important to bear in mind that comedones when they are clearly visible rarely progress to other lesions. It is the ones that are difficult, if not impossible, to see with the naked eye that pose the real threat (see later). The black tops of comedones are not the result of 'ingrained dirt' as promulgated by generations of grandmothers, but are in fact due to melanin. The distinctive site of the blackhead at the tip is a reflection of the microanatomy of the hair follicle.[13] The dominant pathological feature of skin bearing acne lesions is inflammation. The type, density and exact site of the inflammatory cell infiltrate depend on the acuity and severity of the process. The inflammation starts off around the hair follicles and involves the walls of the follicles themselves. The inflammatory cells are both polymorphonuclear leukocytes and mononuclears – predominantly lymphocytes. In older lesions the walls of the follicles are completely disrupted and often only fragments of follicular epithelium are seen. It is thought that the follicle has 'exploded', leaving remnants of follicular debris in the dermis (Figure 4.13). Large numbers of epithelioid cells and foreign body giant cells are evident around these fragments and new fibrous scar tissue can be seen in sheets and bands crossing the scene of devastation (Figures 4.14 and 4.14a).

Aetiopathogenesis

Acne is not due to poor personal hygiene, a 'wild' lifestyle or a poor diet with lots of chocolate. These are folk myths that censorious parents may be sorry to lose. Acne patients, however; seem quite relieved at our current relaxed attitudes.

Inheritance

The question is often asked – is acne inherited? It is such a common disorder that it is very difficult to be certain whether there is a genetic component or not. Many do believe that hereditary factors play an important role but strong evidence is not as yet forthcoming. All ethnic types seem

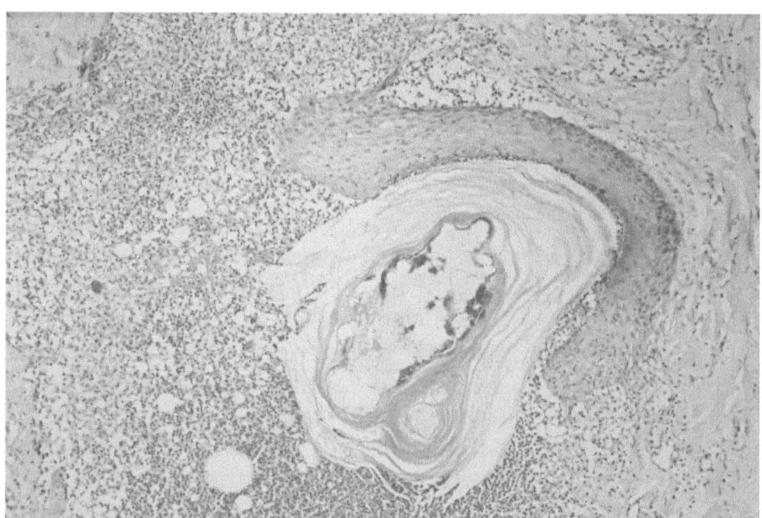

Figure 4.13

Photomicrograph showing ruptured hair follicle from inflamed acne lesion (hematoxylin and eosin × 45).

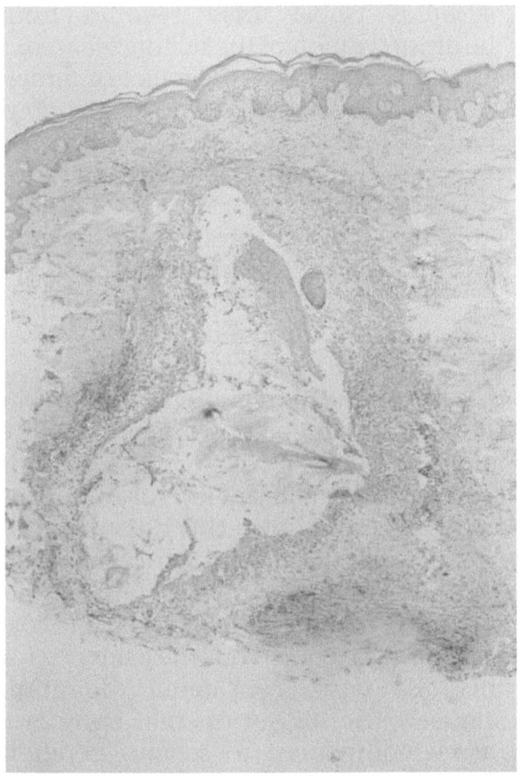

Figure 4.14

Inflammation due to release of follicular contents into dermis (hematoxylin and eosin × 45).

to be affected by acne but there may be as yet uncharacterized national differences in the relative prevalence of the disease. Of course dietetic differences could also account for the latter (see later).

In one report, twin studies[14] indicated a 'substantial genetic influence'. A more recent study of first-degree relatives of patients with persisting facial acne indicated that familial factors determined individual susceptibility. It would be surprising were genetic factors to play no role in any aspect of the disease but it would be equally surprising if the disease was later discovered to be inherited in some Mendelian fashion.

Dietetic factors

Whatever else is true, blaming an 'unhealthy' diet has been part of acne folklore from time immemorial. To quote from an excellent review of the subject;[15] 'This was essentially the Magna Carta for dermatologists of the 1950s; anything coveted by the teenage palate was suspect ....'. As hinted at previously there is

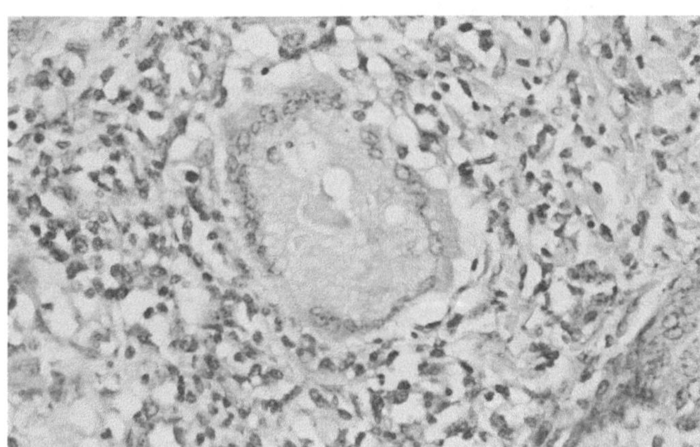

Figure 4.14a

There is an area of inflammatory cell infiltrate in this photomicrograph with a giant cell centrally in response to the release of follicular content into the dermis (hematoxylin and eosin × 120).

anecdotal evidence that some isolated primitive groups of native peoples (such as the Inuit[16] or Kenyan Miral villagers[17]) have very little acne until they start altering their diet to Western foods but overall there is little evidence that diet plays any substantial role in the development of acne. Similarly there are very few well-controlled intervention studies which support a role for food in the genesis of acne. Classical studies in which chocolate has been fed to patients with acne have not succeeded in aggravating the disease[17,18] although such studies have not been beyond criticism. However, a recent, apparently well-controlled study of a 'low glycemic load diet' significantly reduced facial acne compared to a control group. This study should be considered the exception and in general we do not believe at this point that diet is responsible for altering sebum or causing or aggravating acne.

Sebum secretion

Sebum is the unique product of the sebaceous gland consisting of a mixture of lipids (Table 4.1). It arises from the disintegration of the mature sebaceous gland cell and reaches the follicular lumen via the short sebaceous duct as a viscous fluid. Its function is not clear but it has been variously supposed to act as a moisturizer for the skin, to act as a waterproofing lubricant for skin and hair, to have antimicrobial properties and to have no function. In the follicular lumen it is partially hydrolyzed by the lipases of the *Propionibacterium acnes* population so that its composition is altered on the skin surface and is then known as skin surface lipid. The drive to sebum production is provided by the ambient level of androgens and as far as is known this is the major if not the only stimulus to sebaceous gland hyperplasia and sebum secretion. It was suspected that alpha-MSH has some role in sebum secretion[19] but the evidence for this is now considered doubtful. Similarly the suggestion that there is a neural component to sebum secretion has not been substantiated. There is a high density of androgen receptors in the sebaceous glands and testosterone is activated in the follicular apparatus by

TABLE 4.1 Constituents of sebum and skin surface lipid

	'PURE SEBUM'(%)	SKIN SURFACE LIPID(%)
Triglycerides	57	42
Free fatty acids	0	15
Wax esters	25	25
Squalene	15	15
Cholesterol esters	2	2
Cholesterol	1	1

Taken from Leyden JJ. New understandings of the pathogenesis of acne. J Am Acad Dermatol 1995; 32: 815–25.

an enzyme known as 5-alpha-reductase. The conversion of testosterone to 5-dihydrotestosterone appears to be a vital step in the expression of androgenic effects.

Sebum is an essential link in the pathogenesis of acne. There is a linear relationship between the rate of sebum secretion and the severity of the acne,[5] and furthermore, administration of isotretinoin greatly reduces the rate of sebum secretion before improving the acne. Yet sebum clearly is not the only causative agency. Acne develops after exposure to lubricating and cutting oil locally, after exposure to the dioxins systemically and in comedone nevus – in none of which is there any recorded change in the rate of sebum secretion.

Comedones and follicular keratinization

Acne is essentially a folliculitis and it is a common belief that follicular obstruction by comedones is a preliminary prerequisite for acne lesions to develop. Comedones (blackheads) are composed of compacted horn cells and inspissated sebum. The blackened tip is the result of melanin deposition and is a reflection of the position of melanocytes in the external root sheath. Why horn sticks at the mouth of the follicle rather than being shed as it is normally is a mystery and ultimately the major reason for the inflamed lesions of acne.

A study of the ultrastructure of the follicular apparatus in acne demonstrated lipid droplets in the keratinocytes at the neck of the follicle[20] perhaps suggesting a localized abnormality in keratinization. Other explanations for the hyperkeratosis at the mouth of the follicle and comedone formation include the suggestion that there is a functional deficiency in essential fatty acids (linoleic acid in particular) as a result of the differential concentration of different lipid classes at different points within the follicle.[21] While this explanation is interesting and ingenious there is no direct evidence to support it.

Visible comedones rarely provoke inflamed acne lesions; it is those that are too small to be seen – the microcomedones – that are the villains. It is the follicular obstruction caused by these that starts off the cascade of events causing the inflamed lesions of acne.

The microflora

The resident follicular microflora include *Staphylococcus epidermidis*, the yeast *Malassezia furfur* and *P. acnes*. The first two are believed to have no, or at least a trivial, role in the pathogenesis of acne. *P. acnes* – the prolific Gram-positive microaerophilic, lipophilic rod- like microbe – seems to be of major importance in the story. The evidence for its complicity is that its population is greatly increased in acne, acne improves when patients are treated with appropriate antibiotics[22] and some rather neat experiments in which *P. acnes* were injected into cysts in vivo.[23] But how it slots into the overall pathogenetic scheme is by no means clear.

P. acnes is not obviously pathogenic in the same way that *S. aureus* is – so that you can't 'catch acne' from someone with the disease. But *P. acnes* does secrete some potent and potentially important molecules including lipases and proteases, cytokines and mediators. In addition it seems that different strains may have different effects on keratinocytes of the hair follicle modulating their chemokine and antimicrobial peptide expression.[23] *P. acnes* also appears to have an important immunoadjuvant effect which may well be important in modulating the inflammation in acne.[24]

Acne inflammation

Most of the discomfort, disability and distress from acne is due to the inflamed lesions of acne and unfortunately we are a long way from fully understanding the process. Whether inflammation-producing substances diffuse through the follicle wall or follicular contents reach the dermis via cracks in the wall or whether both processes occur together is uncertain. Recent studies have shown that Toll-like receptors show enhanced expression in acne lesions and *P. acnes* triggers inflammatory cytokine responses in acne.[25]

Differential diagnosis

The differential diagnosis includes any disorder in which papules are the presenting lesions and may be mistaken for acne. However, the presence of comedones and seborrhea are strongly supportive of the diagnosis of acne. The absence of signs of other disorders and the presence of scars are also helpful. Table 4.2 lists the main diagnoses to be considered.

Clinical assessment

It is important in all spheres of medicine to attempt to measure the severity and

TABLE 4.2 Differential diagnosis of acne

DISORDER	MAIN DISTINGUISHING FEATURES
Rosacea	No comedones, cysts or scars in rosacea and only face affected
Perioral dermatitis	Micropapules and pustules in nasolabial folds and periorally. Occasionally paranasally and even periocularly. Minimal erythema
Acne agminata	Fixed brownish-red papules on face and upper trunk. No comedones. Leaves scars. Recalcitrant to reatment
Plane warts	Small flat pink-white papules. No comedones or inflamed lesions
Sycosis barbae	Uniform inflamed papules and papulopustules in shaving areas – particularly neck

extent of disease. It is only by using some such measurement technique that the superiority or otherwise of a treatment can be determined both for the individual patient and for groups of patients in the context of clinical trials. By adopting a practical system of measurement it is also possible to learn about correlations between the different clinical phenomena of the disease and between clinical phenomena and laboratory data. Unfortunately it is particularly difficult to arrive at a convenient system of measurement for acne. The variety of clinical lesions and the multiplicity of anatomical sites affected make it difficult to devise a usable method. Purely clinical systems have been quite popular – such as the Leeds Acne Grading System in which standardized photographs are employed for comparison purposes.[26] The difficulties are that identical photographs must be used by all assessors, that there must be consistency in the comparison process and that the grading is arbitrary and non-linear. Recently improvements in photographic technique, for example employing polarized light, has greatly improved our ability to accurately record changes in the skin. Regrettably these improvements do not help in quantifying the abnormalities present.

Clearly some more objective method would be useful but it has been difficult to develop one. An image analysis technique has been used[27] and in a preliminary study seemed to yield promising quantitative data. Unfortunately the system was not developed commercially and has not been used subsequently. The present author has used another system based on the siascopy principle.[28] Essentially, siascopy is a spectroscopic system in which reflected light, in particular wave bands, is assessed quantitatively, enabling the amounts of blood within the skin at various sites to be displayed and measured. A 'non-contact' version of the siascope was employed and in a small group of acne patients measurements made with the siascope correlated well with clinical assessments.

The treatment of acne

The treatment of acne should be early, enthusiastic, pragmatic and optimistic. Acne is a depressing disease and patients need to be encouraged and told in no uncertain terms that they will improve – if the first lot of treatment does not help, then a subsequent one will. It is my practice to prescribe both topical and systemic treatments as this often achieves rather more impressive results than using just one agent at a time. Attacking two of the pathogenetic processes at the same time may be more effective than a single treatment. In general treatments are aimed at one or several of the underlying pathogenetic processes:

- removing the keratinous obstructions at the mouth of the follicles (comedolytics)
- reducing the rate of sebum secretion, either by reducing the androgen drive to sebum secretion (anti-androgens) or by affecting the sebaceous glands themselves (sebotrophic agents)
- reducing the follicular microflora (antimicrobials)
- anti-inflammatory agents.

Topical treatments

Topical retinoids

The topical retinoids include tretinoin (all-*trans*-retinoic acid), isotretinoin, retinaldehyde, adapalene and tazarotene. Retinol (vitamin A) is itself weakly effective as are its esters such as retinyl acetate and retinyl palmitate. Topical retinoids have a powerful comedolytic effect and may also have an anti-inflammatory action. Tretinoin is used at 0.01%, 0.025%, 0.05% and in some countries 0.1% concentrations in lotions, creams and gels. Tretinoin has been available for nearly half a century and remains an important and effective agent for mild to moderate acne.[29] A drawback is the irritation that it may cause. Isotretinoin is likewise a useful topical preparation.[30] The newer synthetic retinoids adapalene[31,32] and tazarotene[33] are both effective to the extent of 60–70% improvement in about 75% of patients within a 6-week period of use. They tend to be more successful in patients without deep nodular or nodulocystic lesions. They are also more suitable for patients whose skin is not easily irritated – some individuals are very susceptible to the irritating effects of topical retinoids and simply cannot tolerate them. They are sometimes formulated with other types of agent such as antibiotics (e.g. isotretinoin with erythromycin – Isotrexin (Stiefel)).

Antimicrobial agents

Benzoyl peroxide

Benzoyl peroxide is one of the oldest topical agents used in the treatment of acne and despite the advent of newer quite useful agents it has maintained a role and some popularity in the treatment of mild forms of the disease. It is mostly formulated as 2, 5 or 10% lotions, gels or creams. It has an antimicrobial effect – particularly on the follicular population of *P. acnes* as these microbes are micro-aerophilic and susceptible to peroxides. Benzoyl peroxide does, however, also have a comedolytic action.

It is certainly suitable for superficial acne but is not as effective as the topical retinoids. It causes irritation of the skin in 10–15% of patients, but rarely may also cause allergic contact hypersensitivity. In addition it bleaches the hair and dyed materials such as textiles with which it comes into contact. Patients must be warned of this effect. Preparations containing benzoyl peroxide are available both as prescription items and as preparations available over the counter at the pharmacy. Benzoyl peroxide is also available in combinations with erythromycin[33] and with clindamycin as gels.[34] There is some therapeutic advantage to these combined formulations as there is greater efficacy than with either agent alone.

Azelaic acid

Azelaic acid is a complex fatty acid and a 'natural product' in that it is produced by the yeast micro-organism that is both a normal inhabitant of the follicles and also responsible for the condition known as pityriasis versicolor (*M. furfur*). It is used in concentrations of 20% in the treatment of acne but 15% for the treatment of rosacea (see page 25). It is thought to act as an antibacterial agent but seems also to have anti-inflammatory actions.[35] It has been reported to have free radical scavenging activity and to slow epidermal differentiation – which may reduce the formation of comedones. In addition it has a depigmentary effect and is used in the treatment of melasma.

It is useful for patients with mild and superficial acne. Azelaic acid gel and cream formulations are well accepted by patients and have a low toxicity without significant adverse side effects.

Other topical antimicrobials

Salicyclic acid in 2% concentration has been used over many years as a component of topical medications for acne. It has antimicrobial and comedolytic actions.

Potassium hydroxyquinoline, the imidazoles (such as miconazole) and the quaternany ammonium compounds have all been used in topical preparations for their antimicrobial effects to treat acne.

Topical antibiotics

The antibiotics used topically in the treatment of acne include erythromycin, tetracycline and clindamycin. They reduce the population of *P. acnes* within the follicle and may also have a variety of anti-inflammatory effects.[36] Topical erythromycin (4%) is the most effective of these giving some 60–65% clinical improvement at around 4–6 weeks after starting treatment. The advantage of topical antibiotics is that they cause little in the way of side effects and are certainly much less irritating than the retinoids and benzoyl peroxide. The major disadvantage of their use is the emergence of resistant strains of *P. acnes* with the ability to transfer that resistance to other microbial species.[37] The emergence of antibiotic resistance certainly appears responsible for escape from treatment control[38] but other more serious consequences are possible but as yet not recorded. The topical antibiotics are also available as combinations with benzoyl peroxide, isotretinoin and tretinoin. These are quite popular with patients and are certainly quite effective.

Other topical agents

Inflammation plays a central role in the clinical manifestations of acne and it is surprising that topical anti-inflammatory agents have not been more extensively explored than they have for their potential usefulness in the management of acne. There is only one licensed product in the UK promoted specifically for its anti-inflammatory action in acne at the time of writing – 4% nicotinamide gel.

Abrasive agents, consisting of minute silica particles are used to assist in comedone removal. They certainly stimulate epidermal proliferation[39] but their success in comedolysis and in the treatment of acne is not well characterized.

Sulfur was at one time a popular component of topical preparations for acne. Although it has fallen out of fashion it is in my experience a safe and effective agent worthy of use in patients with recalcitrant acne. It has comedolytic and antimicrobial properties when used in concentrations of 2–5% in a 'shake' lotion or cream. It can cause some skin irritation and may be associated with unpleasant sulfurous 'rotten eggs' odor.

Systemic treatments

The systemic treatments available include the antibiotics, the retinoids, the anti-androgens and anti-inflammatory agents. They are employed either as second-line agents when topicals are not effective or as first-line agents when it is not practical to use topicals (e.g. when extensive areas of skin are affected). They are often employed alongside topical agents for added efficacy.

Systemic antibiotics

The antibiotics employed include the tetracyclines, erythromycin, clindamycin and trimethoprim/sulfonamide combinations. These latter two are not much used and it is doubtful whether their efficacy/toxicity ratio justifies their use in acne for any other than the rare occasion. They will not be discussed further.

The tetracyclines

The tetracyclines used include tetracycline, oxytetracycline, chlortetracycline, minocycline, doxycycline and lymecycline. The latter three are 'long-acting' and have the strong advantages of needing only to be given once or twice daily and having greater efficacy than the older agents. The tetracyclines suppress the populations of *P. acnes* and the resident micrococci of the pilosebaceous follicles reducing their production of potentially inflammatory products. In addition these agents have important anti-inflammatory actions which aid their therapeutic effects. Some 70% of patients with moderately severe papular acne benefit significantly from administration of the tetracyclines. Improvement begins some 3–4 weeks after starting treatment and the degree of improvement increases over the subsequent 8 weeks or so becoming stabilized with no further improvement at 16 weeks. Dosage regimens vary but it is advisable to start with 'full dosage' and only reduce after the condition has stabilized. The drug should be given until either no further improvement has occurred or no new lesions have appeared in recent weeks.

Adverse side effects are uncommon – the most frequently being minor gastrointestinal disturbances. Some increase in sensitivity to the sun amounting to photosensitivity in some cases is quite common and patients should be warned of the possibility of severe sunburn after relatively trivial sun exposure. Other much less common cutaneous side effects include erythema multiforme and fixed drug eruption. A more serious but uncommon side effect is benign intracranial hypertension marked by headache and ocular disturbances requiring immediate attention. The tetracyclines are teratogenic and must not be used in pregnancy. In addition they are deposited in enamel of developing teeth and cause dental maldevelopment. For this reason they should not be administered to patients below the age of 18 years. There are specific adverse side effects from minocycline administration. The first of these is hyperpigmentation[40] seen either in acne scars, on sun-exposed sites or acrally on the fingers. The brown/black marks develop after the drug has been given for a year or more and unfortunately does not seem to be easily reversible. A more serious problem is a type of hypersensitivity LE-like symptom complex[41,42] in which patients may develop pneumonitis, nephritis, hepatitis or arthritis. This requires immediate withdrawal of the minocycline and institution of treatment with appropriate anti-inflammatory agents.

Overall the most effective, most convenient and least toxic tetracycline would appear to be doxycyline with lymecycline as an alternative.

Erythromycin

Erythromycin is a macrolide antibiotic that is frequently used in patients with inflamed papular lesions of acne. It is employed at a dose of 1 g/day in divided doses and is about as effective as the tetracyclines.[36] The time course of its efficacy is similar to that of the tetracyclines (see above). It is well tolerated with few adverse side effects apart from minor gastrointestinal upset. A major disadvantage of its use is the frequency of induction of erythromycin resistance in *P. acnes*. After a few weeks of use, some 40% of *P. acnes* isolated from the skin are erythromycin-resistant.[43] Microbial resistance usually indicates clinical resistance so that this is not only of theoretical interest but of practical importance as well. It is thought that erythromycin acts in a similar manner to the tetracyclines, i.e. by both suppressing the population of *P. acnes* and as an anti-inflammatory agent.

Anti-androgens

Endogenous androgens provide the drive to sebum production in both men and women and opposing the androgenic action results in a decreased sebum production and hence improvement in the severity of acne. Such anti-androgen treatment interferes with male secondary sex characteristics and depresses sexual function in men. For this reason this type of treatment is only suitable for women. The available licensed agent in the UK containing an anti-androgen is a hormone combination containing the anti-androgen cyproterone acetate (2 mg) and the estrogen ethinyl estradiol (35 μg) (Diane-35). This acts as an oral contraceptive agent though it is only licensed for the treatment of hirsutism, the polycystic ovary syndrome and acne. This combination treatment has been employed in Europe since the 1980s and there is adqequate evidence of the efficacy, acceptability and safety of this agent. Miller et al,[44] for example, in a study of three regimens in 90 subjects, found that the cyproterone acetate and estrogen combination was more effective than standard oral contraceptive therapy. A not dissimilar conclusion was reached by Carlborg in a report of a large multicenter study.[45] The Leeds group found that the combination endocrine treatment was as effective as tetracycline and that it suppressed sebum secretion by 25%.[46] The reduction in skin greasiness noticed by patients after 2 or 3 months on therapy with the cyproterone combination is a bonus but unfortunately there is also a downside. Patients often complain of headaches on the anti-androgen treatment but this is a minor problem compared to the increased risk of thromboembolism in those on the agent. In one study it was found that compared to normal non-pregnant women there was an adjusted odds ratio of 7:44

for venous thrombosis[47] and 2:58 in comparison with those taking conventional oral contraceptives. However, the same group of researchers could not find an increased risk for liver disorders in those taking the anti-androgen preparation.

Other anti-androgens have been tried for acne and it is more than possible that one or another will emerge as a standard treatment. The oldest of these is spironolactone – an aldosterone antagonist and anti-androgen. A report of the published studies to date in a Cochrane Database review[48] concluded that spironolactone 100 mg/day over 6 months produced both objective and subjective improvement in hair growth in patients with hirsutism compared to placebo. However, no conclusion could be reached about the effect in acne as the numbers were too small. Finasteride is a more recently introduced peripherally acting anti-androgen which has been found to be effective in female pattern alopecia and hirsutism. Its activity in acne is as yet uncertain. Flutamide is a further anti-androgen that has been used experimentally via the topical route. At the time of writing anti-androgen treatment is only suitable for women and only indicated for those whose acne is not responding to topical agents and systemic antibiotics. It is particularly useful for patients whose acne is one sign of PCOS.

Systemic isotretinoin (13-*cis* retinoic acid)

The striking efficacy of systemic isotretinoin (a retinoid) in severe cystic acne was discovered fortuitously during exploratory treatment with isotretinoin of patients with severe disorders of keratinization who also had cystic acne.[49] It became evident early on that isotretinoin was an extremely potent drug capable of controlling cystic acne – a disease for which there had been no effective treatment previously. Early studies demonstrated that this retinoid greatly reduced the rate of sebum secretion.[50] Oral administration of isotretinoin seemed to shrivel the sebaceous glands but how it did this has never been entirely clear – made even more difficult to understand by the fact that other retinoids did not seem to possess this activity. Recently experimental work[51] has been reported that suggests that this action of isotretinoin is in fact not retinoid receptor-mediated and appears to depend on activation of 'apoptotic pathways' within sebaceous gland cells.

It is not even certain whether it is isotretinoin itself or one of its metabolites (all-*trans*-retinoic acid, 9-*cis* retinoic acid, 4-oxo-retinoic acid, etc.) that is responsible for its pharmacological effects. It seems likely that anti-inflammatory effects also play a role in the mode of action.

Indications

When first introduced in 1982/1983 dermatologists were unfamiliar with isotretinoin and fearful of its potential for unpleasant adverse side effects; the recommendation was that it was only used for patients with severe recalcitrant cystic acne. Some 20 years later all seemed to agree that isotretinoin should be prescribed for a wider group of patients including those with less severe acne that is causing or probably will cause scarring and those with severe psychological stress as a result of acne.[52,53] Those with 'resistant' and recurrent disease also now qualify for treatment with isotretinoin.

Dose and length of treatment

The recommended length of a course of treatment is 4–6 months and studies have shown that a total cumulated dose of 120–150 mg/kg is associated with the lowest recurrence rate.[54] From this it follows that a daily dose of 0.5–1 mg/kg is the best in the longer term. Claims that patients do very well on a low-dose regimen have been made – one study contrasted patients with a low dose (0.15–0.4 mg/kg/day) with another group treated with the usual 0.5–1.0 mg/kg/day and found a success rate of 69% in the low-dose group and a reduced incidence of adverse side effects.[55] However, the same minimum total dose of 120 mg/kg needs to be achieved to prevent relapses – should the response be inadequate a further course should be given after a 4-week gap.

Efficacy

At the end of the course of treatment more than 90% of patients should be clear of acne lesions. Most of those who are given a second course because of an inadequate response to the first course do respond. Quite frequently there is an initial aggravation of the acne. Some 30–40% of patients experience an outbreak of new acne lesions as well as a worsening of the inflamed lesions already present. Reduction of the severity of acne usually starts some 8–10 weeks after the start of treatment and continues from there on.

Adverse side effects

Teratogenicity

Retinol and all retinoids have profound teratogenic effects when administered during fetal development. Serious cardiac, CNS, renal, skeletal and craniofacial defects occur in fetuses when they are exposed to isotretinoin during early pregnancy. Precise figures have been difficult to collect but it may be expected that 25% of pregnancies during which isotretinoin has been given orally may be expected to end in severe malformation, while 50% end in spontaneous abortion.[56] To avoid such a tragic outcome the following measures should be adopted:

- patient education by discussion and pamphlets
- pregnancy testing before starting treatment and repeating the test after 1 month
- the use of two methods of contraception in *all* fertile women
- avoidance of pregnancy for 1 month after stopping treatment.

Lipid abnormalities

Hypertriglyceridemia and hypercholesterolemia occur in 25% of patients on isotretinoin.[57] This usually returns to normal after stopping treatment but care is needed for patients with atherosclerosis and lipid disorders. Blood monitoring for lipid levels before and during the treatment is mandatory. It is prudent to advise a reduction in the fat content of the diet for patients whose blood lipids increase.

Liver abnormalities

A moderate elevation of the transaminases occurs in some 15% patients.[58] The elevation settles quickly after treatment stops. True drug-induced hepatitis does occur but it is extremely rare.[55] Blood monitoring for transaminase levels before and during treatment is mandatory.

Bone abnormalities

It was well known that vitamin A caused skeletal abnormalities in experimental animals as, in fact, it was found subsequently did the retinoid drugs. It was, therefore, no surprise that reports of bony changes in patients taking the retinoid drugs started to appear in the mid to late 1980s. The large majority of these have been discovered by radiological survey or by chance and have been asymptomatic. Most of the reports have been of hyperostosis of the vertebrae (e.g. references 59 and 60) and have simulated the spontaneously occurring condition known as disseminated interstitial skeletal hyperostosis. More worrying is the case reports of ossification of the posterior longitudinal spinal ligament.[61] Clearly dysfunction due to pressure on spinal column tracts is a distinct possibility in such patients.

Various other bony abnormalities have been claimed but have not been confirmed. Premature epiphyseal closure, for example, has been of concern but not clinically proven.

Psychiatric abnormalities

Major concerns have been expressed over the association between the administration of isotretinoin and the development of depression, attempted suicide and suicide. The major difficulty is that acne itself causes depression and suicide in adolescence is not uncommon. Systematic reviews did not reveal a specific epidemiologic association between isotretinoin and depression.[62,63] There is however, 'case report evidence' that 'isotretinoin may be associated with the development of depression'. Furthermore, a brain imaging study employing positron emission tomography demonstrated that a group of acne patients taking isotretinoin had decreased brain metabolism in the orbitofrontal cortex – a brain area known to mediate depression as compared to patients on antibiotics.[64] It seems that although the door leading to the relationship between isotretinoin and depression is shut – it is by no means locked. Acne patients should be checked for depression before isotretinoin is started.

Mucocutaneous side effects

Unlike the above adverse side effects virtually all on the drug experience these to a greater or lesser extent. Cheilitis – or at least dry lips – is uncomfortable but can be eased with regular use of white soft paraffin (Figure 4.15). Drying of the nasal mucosa often leads to nose bleeds and dry sore eyes may make the wearing of contact lenses difficult. If severe the drying can lead to a facial dermatitis

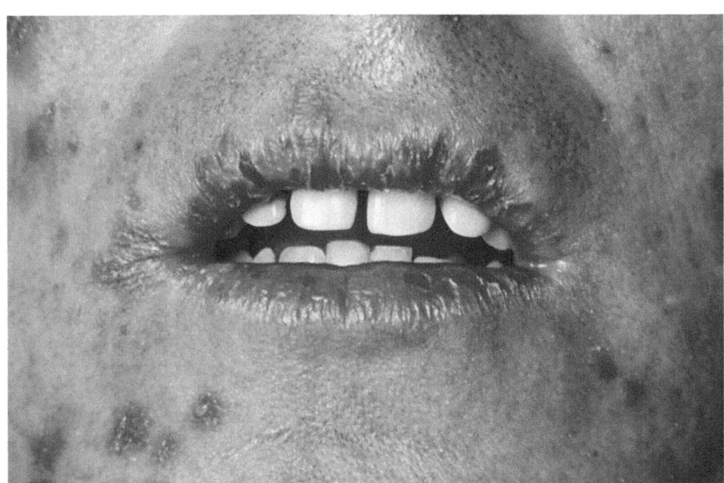

Figure 4.15

Dry cracked lips (cheilitis) – this is commonly seen after starting isotretinoin by mouth. It rapidly resolves when the course is finished.

requiring emollients and even weak corticosteroids.

Miscellaneous adverse side effects

Myalgia is a frequent complaint but is in general not a disabling symptom. Arthralgia is also an occasional problem. A curious but well-documented side effect is the development of paronychiae (Figure 4.16). The development of pyogenic granuloma-like lesions is probably related to these paronychiae.

Intracranial hypertension causing headaches, papilloedema and ocular problems is a rare result of isotretinoin administration. The results of a survey in the USA established the association and recorded 179 instances of this side effect.[65]

Alopecia

A small proportion of patients taking isotretinoin (perhaps 15–20%) complain of increased shedding of scalp hair and the appearance of 'thinning' of the hair.

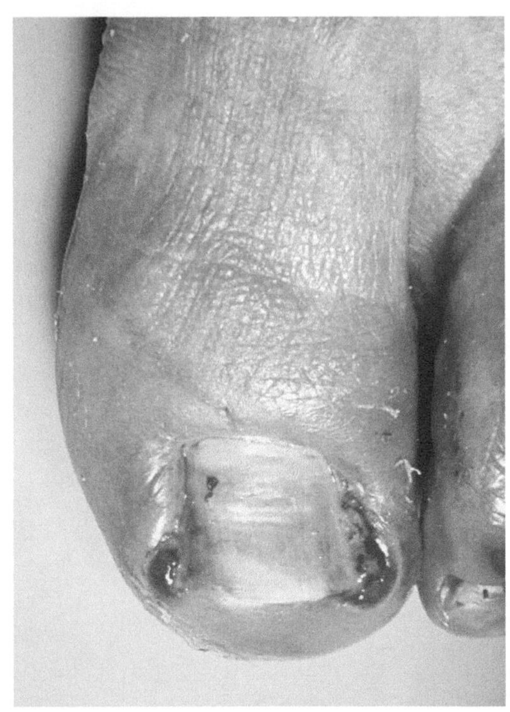

Figure 4.16

Paronychiae. This is a side effect of isotretinoin administration.

Luckily the hair returns to normal in most patients after stopping the drug. The mechanism of this problem is uncertain as it does not appear to be the result of anagen arrest as with anticancer drugs or due to telogen effluvium. It has been claimed that hair loss occurring during administration of the aromatic retinoid etretinate is due to what was termed a follicular anchorage defect.[63] It is possible that the hair loss due to isotretinoin is the result of a similar anchorage defect. After the hair loss described above the subsequent regrowth may look different from the original hair in that it may be curly or altered in other ways (Figure 4.17).

Other systemic drugs sometimes used in acne

Dapsone is sometimes employed in individuals with very severe acne who for one reason or another are not responding to standard treatments. Corticosteroids are also employed for patients who have a severe acne flare or who have acne fulminans.

Phototherapy

Anecdotal reports of the beneficial effects of sunlight, real and artificial, in patients with acne vulgaris were commonplace a half century ago, but did not receive serious consideration until the 1990s. Now it is recognized that phototherapy of a wide variety of types can be helpful to patients at various stages of the disease. It seems that photodynamic therapy with topical 5-aminolevulinic or methylaminolevulinic acid can reduce the amount of inflammatory acne present after only two or three treatments.[66] Similarly radiation with blue light from LED sources will also reduce inflammatory acne.[67] Red light has also been used and found helpful. It seems that there are many light sources and modalities that are being used for acne treatment but there is not the same level of confirmatory evidence for all of their usefulness!

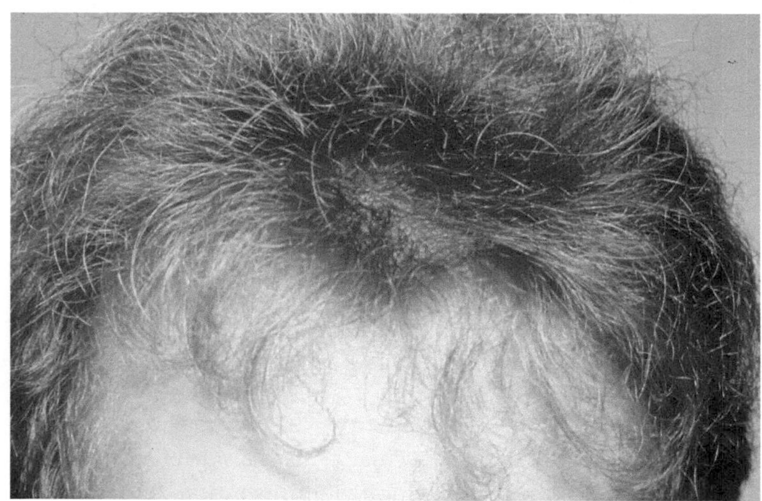

Figure 4.17

Curly hair. This is a rare side effect of isotretinoin treatment.

It should be noted that there are also reports of the use of lasers for the treatment of 'atrophic acne scars'.[68]

References

1. Cunliffe WJ, Gollnick HPM. Acne Diagnosis and Management. London: Martin Dunitz, 2001.
2. Plewig G, Kligman AM. Acne and Rosacea. Berlin: Springer, 2000.
3. Kesseler T, Enderer K, Steigler GK. Quantitative analysis of skin surface lipids using a sebumeter method. Random lipid levels on the skin surface during therapy with 13-cis retinoic acid, minocycline hydrochloride and UVA rays. Z Hautlem 1985; 60: 857–65.
4. Pochi PE, Strauss JS. Sebum production, casual sebum levels, titrable acidity of sebum, and urinary fractional 17 ketosteroid expression in moles with acne. J Invest Dermatol 1964; 43: 383.
5. Cunliffe WJ, Shuster S. Pathogenesis of acne. Lancet 1969; 1: 685–7.
6. Marks R. Acne and its management beyond the age of 35 years. Am J Clin Dermatol 2004; 5: 459–62.
7. Tucker SB, Flannigan SA, Dunbar M Jr et al. Development of an objective comedogenicity assay. Arch Dermatol 1986; 122: 660–5.
8. Mills H, Kligman AM. A human model for assessing comedogenic substances. Arch Dermatol 1982; 118: 903–5.
9. Grant JE, Phillips KA. Recognising and treating body dysmorphic disorder. Ann Clin Psychiatry 2005; 17: 205–10.
10. Buggs C, Rosenfeld RL. Polycystic ovary syndrome in adolescence. Endocrinol Metab Clin North Am 2005; 34: 677–705.
11. Hamburg R. Polycystic ovary syndrome in adolescence. New insights in pathophysiology and treatment. Endocr Dev 2005; 8: 137–49.
12. Schechner S. What is dioxin anyway? Where does it come from? 2005. And are its effects reversible: Internet posted 13 December 2004.
13. Blair G, Lewis CA. The pigment of comedones. Br J Dermatol 1970; 82: 572.
14. Friedman GD. Twin studies of disease heritability based on medical records: application to acne vulgaris. Acta Genet Med Gemellol (Roma) 1984; 33: 487.
15. Wolf R, Matz H, Orion E. Acne and diet. Clin Dermatol 2004; 22: 387–93.
16. Bendiner E. Distastrous trade off: Eskimo health for white "civilizations". Hosp Pract 1974; 9: 156–89.
17. Verhagen A, Koten J, Chaddah V et al. Skin diseases in Kenya. A clinical and histopathological study of 3,168 patients. Arch Dermatol 1968; 98: 577–86.
18. Fulton J, Plewig G, Kligman A. Effect of chocolate on acne vulgaris. JAMA 1969; 210: 2071–4.
19. Goolamali SL, Burton JL, Shuster S. Sebum excretion in hypopituitarism. Br J Dermatol 1973; 89: 21–4.
20. Knutson D. Ultrastructural observations in acne vulgaris. The normal sebaceous follicle and acne lesions. J Invest Dermatol 1974; 6: 288–307.
21. Downing DT, Stewart ME, Wertz PW et al. Essential fatty acids and acne. J Am Acad Dermatol 1986; 14: 221–5.
22. Kurschbaum JD, Kligman AM. The pathogenic role of Propionibacterium acnes in acne vulgaris. Arch Dermatol 1963; 88: 832–3.
23. Nagy I, Pivarcsi A, Kis K et al. Propionibacterium acnes and lipopolysaccharide induce the expression of antimicrobial peptides and proinflammatory cytokines/chemokines in human sebocytes. Microbes Infect 2006; E-pub.
24. Jappe U, Ingham E, Henwood J et al. Propionibacterium acnes and inflammation in acne. P. acnes has T-cell mitogenic activity. Br J Dermatol 2002; 146: 2002–9.
25. Jugeau S, Tenaud I, Knol AC et al. Induction of Toll like receptors by Propionibacterium acnes. Br J Dermatol 2005; 153: 1105–13.
26. O'Brien SG, Lewis JB, Cunliffe WJ. The Leeds revised acne grading system. J Dermatol Treat 1998; 9: 215–220.
27. Friedman PM, Skover GR, Payonk G. Quantitative evaluation of non-ablative laser

technology. Semin Cutan Med Surg 2002; 21: 266–73.

28. Cotton S, Marks R. Accurate machine assessment of acne and rosacea. Paper read at meeting of International Society of Bioengineering and the Skin, Orlando, America, Oct. 2004.
29. Lucky AW, Cullen S, Funicella T et al. Double blind vehicle controlled multicenter comparison of two 0.025% tretinoin creams in patients with acne vulgaris. J Am Acad Dermatol 1998; 38: 524–30.
30. Chalker DK, Lesher JL, Smith JG Jr et al. Efficacy of topical isotretinoin 0.05% gel on acne vulgaris: results of a multicenter double blind investigation. J Am Acad Dermatol 1987; 17: 251–4.
31. Thiboutot DM, Shalita AR, Yamanuchi PS et al. Adapalene gel 0.1% as maintenance therapy for acne vulgaris: a randomized controlled investigator blind follow up of a recent study. Arch Dermatol 2006; 142: 597–602.
32. Shalita A, Miller B, Menter A et al. Tazarotene cream versus adopalene cream in the treatment of facial acne vulgaris: a multicenter double-blind, randomized parallel-group study. J Drugs Dermatol 2005; 4: 153–8.
33. Ozolin SM, Eady EA, Avery AJ et al. Comparison of five antimicrobial regimens for treatment of mild to moderate inflammatory facial acne vulgaris in the community: randomized clinical trial. Lancet 2004; 364: 2188–95.
34. Bowman S, Gold M, Nasir A et al. Comparison of clindamycin, benzoyl peroxide, tretinoin plus clindamycin and the combination of clindamycin/benzoyl peroxide and tretinoin plus clindamycin in the treatment of acne vulgaris: a randomized blinded study. J Drugs Dermatol 2005; 4: 611–18.
35. Fitton A, Goa KL. Azelaic acid. A review of its pharmacological properties and therapeutic efficacy in acne and hyperpigmentation skin disorders. Drugs 1991; 41: 780–98.
36. Plewig G, Schopf E. Anti-inflammatory effects of antimicrobial agents: an in-vivo study. J Invest Dermatol 1975; 65: 532–6.
37. Leyden J, Levy S. The development of antibiotic resistance in Propionibacterium acnes. Cutis 2001; 67: 21–4.
38. Cunliffe WJ. Propionibacterium acnes resistance and its clinical relevance. J Dermatol Treat 1995; 6 (Suppl 1): 53–4.
39. Marks R, Hill S, Barton SP. The effects of an abrasive agent on normal skin and on photoaged skin in comparison with topical tretinoin. Br J Dermatol 1990; 123: 457–66.
40. Ododuik-Gad RP, Morentim HM, Schafer J et al. Minocycline induced cutaneous hyperpigmentation: confocal laser scanning microscope analysis. J Eur Acad Dermatol Venereol 2006; 20: 435–9.
41. van Steensel MA. Why minocycline can cause systemic lupus erythematosus and suggestions for therapeutic intervention. Med Hypotheses 2004; 63: 31–4.
42. Lawson TM, Amos N, Bulgen D, Williams BD. Minocycline-induced lupus: clinical features and response to rechallenge. Rheumatology (Oxford) 2001; 40: 329–35.
43. Oprica C, Metestam L, Lapins J et al. Antibiotic resistant Propionibacterium acnes on the skin of patients with moderate to severe acne in Stockholm. Anaerobe 2004; 10: 155–64.
44. Miller JA, Wojnarowska FT, David PM et al. Anti-androgen treatment in women with acne: a controlled trial. Br J Dermatol 1986; 114: 705–16.
45. Carlborg L. Cyproterone acetate versus levonorgestrel combined with ethinyl estradiol in the treatment of acne. Results of a multicenter study. Acta Obstet Gynecol Scand Suppl 1986; 134: 29–39.
46. Greenwood R, Brummitt L, Burke BC et al. Acne: double blind clinical and laboratory trial of tetracycline oestrogen cyproterone acetate and combined treatment. Br Med J (Clin Res Ed) 1985; 291: 1231–5.
47. Seamen HE, Vries CS Farmer RD. The risk of thromboembolism in women prescribed cyproterone acetate in combination with ethinyl estradiol: a nested cohort analysis and case control study. Hum Reprod 2003; 18: 522–6.
48. Farquhar C, Lee O, Toomath R, Jepson R. Spironolactone versus placebo or in combination with steroids for hirsutism

and/or acne. Cochrane Database Syst Rev 2003; 4: CD000194.

49. Peck GL, Yoder FW. Treatment of lamellar ichthyosis and other keratinising disorders with an oral synthetic retinoid. Lancet 1976; 27(2): 1172–4.
50. Strauss JS, Stewart ME, Downing DT. The effect of 13-cis-retinoic acid on sebaceous glands. Arch Dermatol 1987; 123: 1538–41.
51. Nelson AM, Gilliland KL, Cong Z, Thiboutot DM. 13-cis retinoic acid induces apoptosis and cell cycle arrest in human SEB-1 sebocytes. J Invest Dermatol 2006; E. pub. ahead of print.
52. Cooper AJ. Treatment of acne with isotretinoin: recommendations based on Australian experience. Aust J Dermatol 2003; 44: 97–105.
53. Goldsmith LA, Bolognia JI, Callen JP et al. American Academy of Dermatology. Consensus conference on the safe and optimal use of isotretinoin: summary and recommendations. J Am Acad Dermatol 2004; 50: 900–6.
54. Layton AM, Stainforth JM, Cunliffe WJ. 10 years' experience of oral isotretinoin for the treatment of acne vulgaris. J Dermatol Treat 1994; 4(Suppl 2): 52–5.
55. Mandekou-Lefaki I, Delli F, Teknetzis A. Low doses scheme of isotretinoin in acne vulgaris. Int J Clin Pharmacol Res 2003; 23: 41–4.
56. Mitchell AA, van Bennekom CM, Louik CA. A pregnancy prevention program in women of childbearing age receiving isotretinoin. N Engl J Med 1995; 333: 101–6.
57. Ellis CN, Krach KJ. Uses and complications of isotretinoin therapy. J Am Acad Dermatol 2001; 45: S150–7.
58. Falton MB, Boyer JL. Hepatic toxicity of vitamin A and synthetic retinoids. J Gastroenterol Hepatol 1990; 5: 332–42.
59. McGuire J, Lawson JP. Skeletal changes associated with chronic isotretinoin and etretinate administration. Dermatologica 1987; 175(Suppl 1): 169–81.
60. Gerber LH, Helfgott RK, Gross EG et al. Vertebral abnormalities associated with synthetic retinoid use. J Am Acad Dermatol 1984; 10: 817–23.
61. Pennes DR, Martel W, Ellis CN. Retinoid induced ossification of the posterior longitudinal ligament. Skeletal Radiol 1985; 14: 191–3.
62. Marqueling AL, Zane LT. Depression and suicidal behaviour in acne patients treated with isotretinoin: a systemic review. Semin Cutan Med Surg 2005; 24: 92–102.
63. Hull PR, D'Arcy C. Acne, depression and suicide. Dermatol Clin 2005; 23: 665–74.
64. Bremner JD, Fani N, Ashraf A et al. Functional brain imaging alterations in acne patients treated with isotretinoin. Am J Psychiatry 2005; 162: 983–91.
65. Fraunfelder FW, Fraunfelder FT, Corbett JJ. Isotretinoin associated intracranial hypertension. Ophthalmology 2004; III: 1248–50.
66. Hongcharu W, Taylor CR, Chang Y et al. Topical ALA photodynamic therapy for the treatment of acne vulgaris. J Invest Dermatol 2000; 115: 183–92.
67. Tzung TY, Wu KH, Huang ML. Blue light phototherapy in the treatment of acne. Photodermatol Photoimmunol Photomed 2004; 20: 266–9.
68. Tanzi EL, Alster TS. Comparison of a 1450-nm diode laser and a 1320-nm Nd: YAG laser in the treatment of atrophic facial scars: a prospective clinical and histologic study. Dermatol Surg 2004; 30: 152–7.

Psoriasis and congenital disorders of keratinization

Psoriasis

It is often stated that this common scaling skin disorder rarely affects the face. Although it is certainly the case that classical psoriasis usually affects the skin of the knees, elbows, lower back and scalp, in my experience the face is all too often affected.

Interestingly, facial psoriasis seems more common in children than in adults.[1] Facial involvement was thought, in one study, to be a marker of severe psoriasis and was found to occur in some 67% of the patients examined.[2]

Clinical features

Typically patches develop on the forehead adjacent to affected scalp skin (Figures 5.1a and 5.1b). Similarly the retro-auricular areas are sometimes involved. Psoriatic lesions occurring at these sites are quite typical for ordinary psoriasis occurring on the skin of the trunk or limbs in that they are red and scaly and the edges are rounded or polycyclic and quite well defined. When psoriasis occurs on the cheeks and neck the edges tend to be more diffuse. As discussed on page 73, there are patients with seborrheic dermatitis who develop lesions that have a very psoriasiform appearance – a situation to

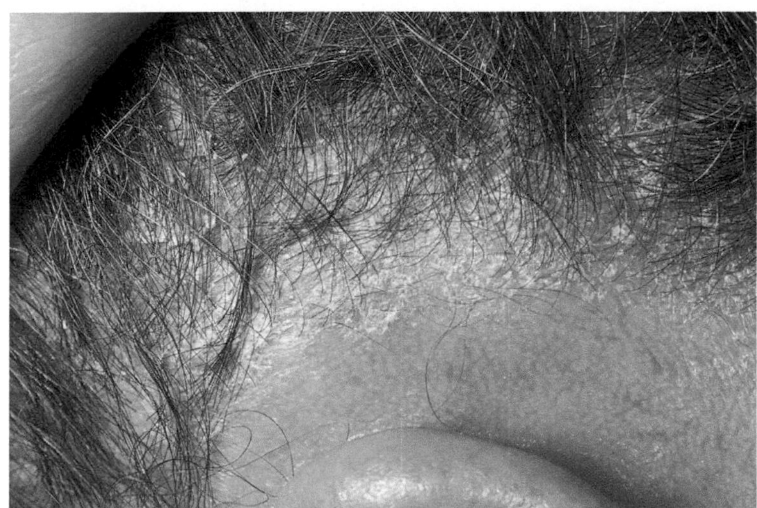

Figure 5.1a

Psoriasis of scalp margin.

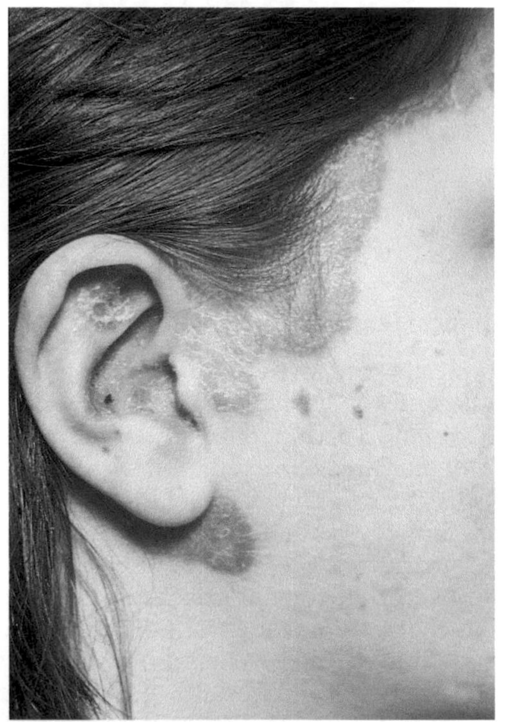

Figure 5.1b

Another example of psoriasis affecting the scalp margin.

which the term 'seborrhiasis' has been applied. This curious condition is marked by red scaling lesions affecting the nasolabial folds, the retroauricular areas and other flexural sites (Figure 5.2). Most forms of facial psoriasis tend to be short-lived or even transient compared to plaques on the limbs or trunk. Even the scalp tends to hang on to its psoriatic patches more stubbornly than does the face.

Uncommonly, in severe generalized psoriasis the face may be uniformly red and the condition is then not easily distinguished as psoriasis. In fact, a number of disorders including drug allergies, and disorders of keratinization can present with a 'red face' and no other distinguishing features making a clinical diagnosis very difficult.[3]

Differential diagnosis

The major diagnostic confusion with facial psoriasis is, as mentioned previously, with seborrheic dermatitis. Nonetheless, most patients can be assigned one or another of these diagnoses by reference

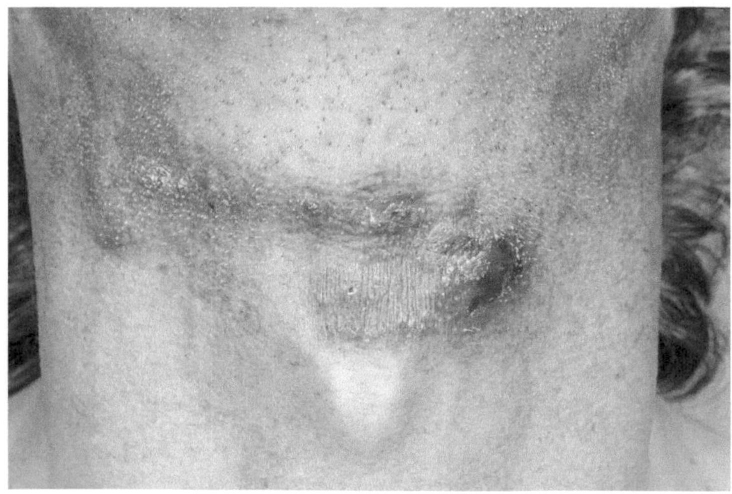

Figure 5.2

Patchy red, scaling areas affecting front of the neck that look psoriasis-like, but are in fact caused by seborrheic dermatitis – so-called 'seborrhiasis'.

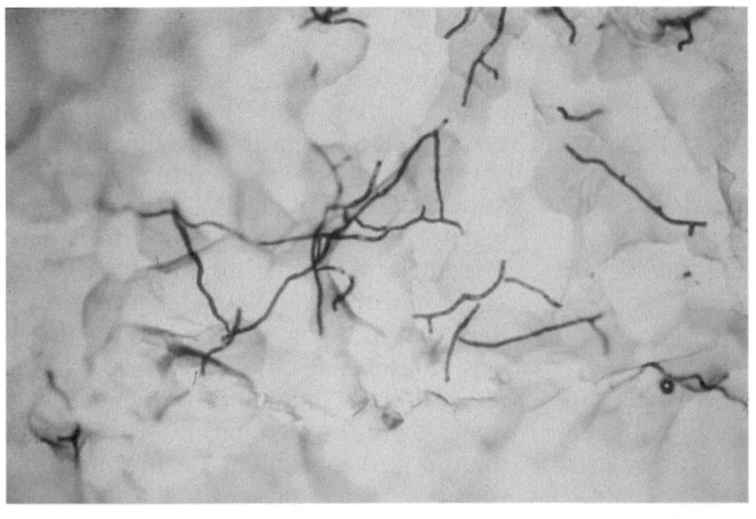

Figure 5.3

Pink/purple fungal mycelium visible in a skin surface biopsy sample taken from patch of ringworm (periodic acid – Schiff reagent stain × 45).

to their history and the presence of skin lesions on the trunk and/or limbs. There are some, though, whose disease defies confident diagnosis and for these I have to admit (reluctantly) that the name seborrhiasis is apt and convenient – even if it only proves to be a temporary pigeon hole.

Ringworm lesions are red, scaling and annular, round or polycyclic but the disease tends to spring suddenly 'out of nowhere', to spread more rapidly and be more inflamed than psoriasis. Ringworm lesions may be solitary or if multiple are not symmetrical as psoriasis usually is. Investigation of the surface scale by either the classic KOH method or preferably the skin surface biopsy method[4] will reveal interlacing fungal mycelium (Figure 5.3).

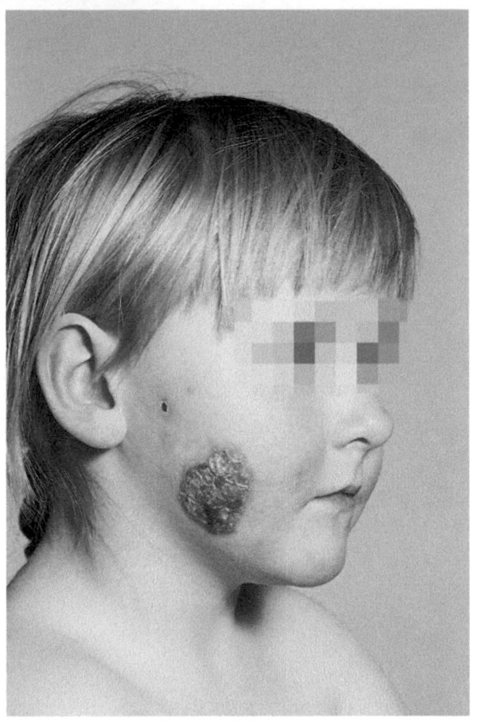

Figure 5.4

Impetigo – sometimes this can have a psoriasis-like appearance.

Another infective disorder that may be confused with psoriasis – and has certainly confused the author on at least one occasion (Figure 5.4) – is impetigo (see Chapter 10). This condition sometimes starts off as red scaling patches and looks quite psoriasis-like. However, untreated impetigo soon declares itself by spreading and by blistering and producing golden-yellow crusted patches.

Discoid lupus erythematosus often produces well-defined red scaling plaques that may superficially simulate psoriasis but their fixity, irregularity in outline, dyspigmentation and scarring should help differentiate these lesions from psoriasis. (see page 115).

Non-melanoma skin cancer including solar keratoses, Bowen's disease and basal cell carcinoma are extremely common in white-skinned Caucasian subjects. For the most part these do not look or behave like psoriasis. Nonetheless, it must be admitted that all the lesions mentioned can occasionally produce well-defined red scaling patches on facial skin (Figure 5.5). Superficial basal cell carcinoma can reach 1–2 cm^2 in size before the patient presents and by that time may look very psoriasiform – the characteristic 'thread-like' margin being subtle and quite unobtrusive. These are quite uncommon on the face. Similarly a patch of Bowen's disease may closely resemble psoriasis. It is worth mentioning that rarely T-cell lymphoma of the skin may present on the face as a solitary psoriasiform patch without particular diagnostic features. Biopsy is needed to establish a diagnosis.

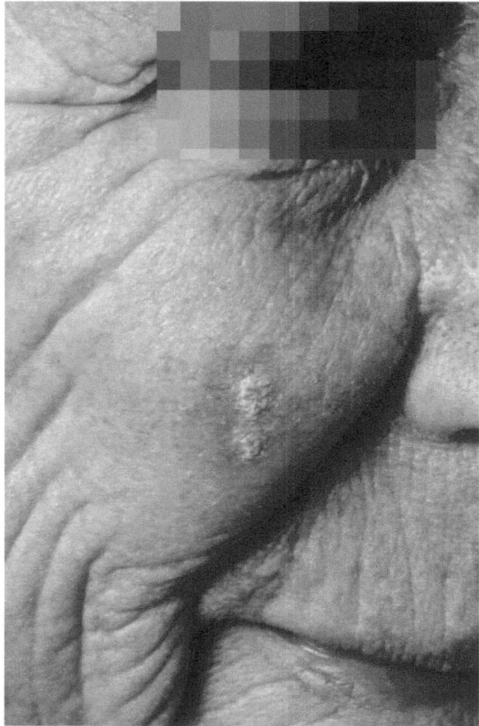

Figure 5.5

Scaling pink patch on face due to solar keratosis.

Ulerythema ophryogenes is a strange, uncommon disorder of unknown origin affecting children 7–15 years of age. Pink scaling areas occur in the eyebrows and over the forehead and cheeks. In addition there is usually marked keratosis pilaris affecting the lateral aspects of the upper arms.

Pathology

The regular epidermal thickening with club-like epidermal down-growths, parakeratosis, suprapapillary thinning, papillary capillary dilation and tortuosity, and Munro microabscess formation of classical plaque-like psoriasis is rarely observed in all its glory in facial psoriasis. Generally, it is a much more muted affair with a variable degree of regular epidermal thickening and some inflammation. The important issue about biopsy of psoriasiform facial lesions is that this maneuver should decisively rule out the sometimes clinically similar disorders such as discoid lupus erythematosus and the various forms of non-melanoma skin cancer.

Treatment

Many of the topical treatments used for psoriasis of the skin of the trunk and limbs are unsuitable for treatment of facial lesions as facial skin is so much more easily irritated. Luckily the facial lesions of most patients with psoriasis respond readily to fairly innocuous treatments with emollients and weak corticosteroids such as 1% hydrocortisone or 0.1% clobetasone butyrate. More stubborn lesions may respond to the careful use of moderately potent or potent topical corticosteroid preparations over limited periods of less than 4 weeks. Fluticasone propionate (0.005%) ointment was used in one study of 20 patients[5] with facial psoriasis. A regimen over a 10-week period proved very successful without causing significant atrophy. Similarly, superpotent topical steroids are often used as adjuncts to systemic therapy for plaque-type psoriasis but according to one group should not be used for facial or flexural psoriasis.[6] Clearly great care must be taken as telangiectasia and the other signs of skin atrophy may rapidly appear on facial skin and once established take a long time to recover. Treatment with the least-potent agent that is effective for the least time should be taken as guidelines. Vitamin D_3 analogs are successful topical treatments for ordinary plaque-type psoriasis (e.g. calcipotriol, tacalcitol, calcitriol). Unfortunately they cause not inconsiderable irritation and great caution must be used when the face is treated. A combination of calcipotriol and betamethasone-17-valerate is available and designed to avoid irritation. Several reports have appeared describing the beneficial results of the use of topical tacrolimus in facial psoriasis. One hundred and sixty-seven patients were evaluated in one 8-week randomized double-blind vehicle controlled study of 0.1% tacrolimus used bd for facial or intertriginous psoriasis. Sixty-five percent of the tacrolimus group were almost clear at 8 weeks compared to 31% of the 'control' patients.[7] Whether systemic treatments are used or not should depend on the overall severity of the disorder as a whole and not just on the facial condition. Drugs such as methotrexate, cyclosporine, the aromatic retinoids and the newer 'biologics' are all effective – but potentially toxic and should only be given after discussion with the patient and drawing up a carefully designed treatment and monitoring plan. Details of such treatments may be found in reference 4.

Pityriasis rubra pilaris (PRP)

This fairly uncommon disease mainly affects the late middle aged and elderly. There is also a quite rare infantile variety which we will not consider any further here. PRP often starts quite abruptly without warning as a pink scaling rash over the face and scalp. The color is quite distinctive having a salmon-pink or orangey hue (Figure 5.6). The rash often spreads onto the trunk and indeed may cause an erythroderma with curious islands of unaffected normal skin. On the back of the fingers, over the front and sides of the thighs, upper arms and buttocks there is the feature that gives PRP its name in which the follicles are

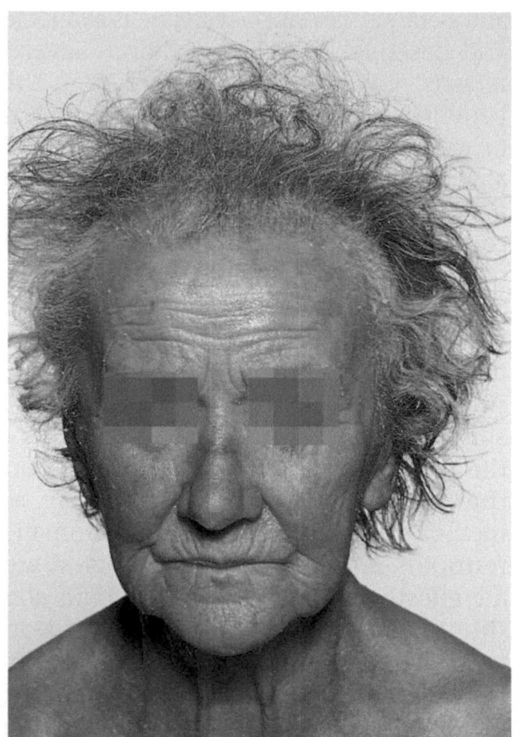

Figure 5.6

This patient has pityriasis rubra pilaris. The rash started on the face and scalp and was of an orangey hive.

pink, prominent and contain a horny plug. The condition tends to remit after 12–18 months but can recur.

Pathology

Marked regular epidermal thickening and parakeratosis characterize the picture. The absence of Munro microabscesses, suprapapillary thinning, the papillary capillary changes and the inflammation of psoriasis help in distinguishing the conditions.

Treatment

Emollients may temporarily improve the appearance and provide some relief from discomfort but do nothing to alter the course of the disease. Systemic methotrexate or aromatic retinoids (acitretin or tazarotene) do have an improving action but generally need to be given over some months before they can be stopped without fear of the disease returning. The side effects of

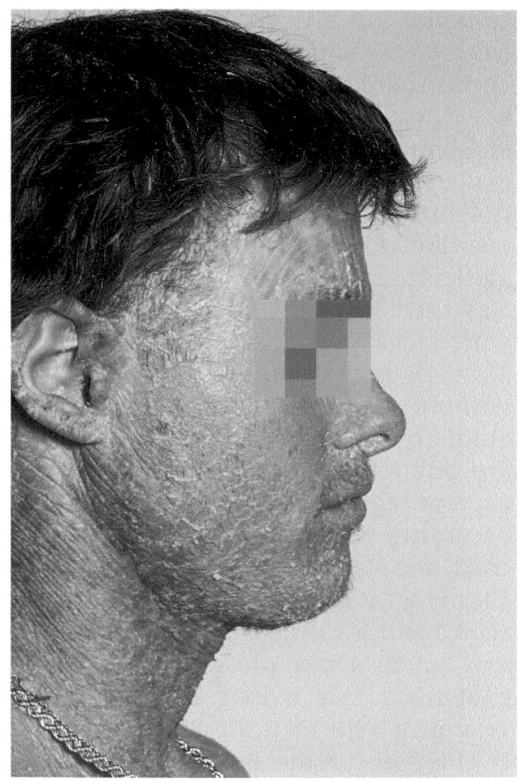

Figure 5.7

This young man has lamellar ichthyosis. This rare recessive disorder causes marked scaling with ectropion and 'crumpled ears'.

both methotrexate and the retinoids are frequent and may cause serious harm.

Congenital disorders of keratinization

In the rare recessive disorder lamellar ichthyosis the ears have a 'crumpled' appearance and there is an accompanying and disfiguring ectropion (Figure 5.7). These signs are not specific to lamellar ichthyosis but are seen to a lesser extent in other severe congenital scaling disorders and may be due to fetal facial development being disturbed by the presence of rigid inelastic stratum corneum. The skin of the cheeks, forehead and neck is dry and scaling.

Typically in sex-linked ichthyosis and occasionally in severe autosomal dominant ichthyosis the sides of the neck and to a lesser extent the sides of the face show a marked scaliness, the surface being broken up into large brown lamellae.

Face skin is also affected by pinkness and fine scaling in non-bullous ichthyosiform erythroderma and in some types of erythrokeratoderma variablis.

References

1. Farber EM. Facial psoriasis. Cutis 1992; 50: 25–8.
2. Park JY, Rim JH, Choe YB et at. Facial psoriasis. J Am Acad Dermatol 2004; 50: 582–4.
3. Schuster Ch, Burg G. The red face. Schweitz Ruøidsch Med Prax 2004; 93: 1727–32.
4. Marks, R Dawber RPR. In situ microbiology of the stratum corneum. Arch Dermatol 1972; 105: 216–21.
5. Lebwohl MG, Tan MH, Meador SL et al. Limited application of fluticasone propionate ointment, 0.005% in patients with psoriasis of the face and intertriginous areas. J Am Acad Dermatol 2001; 44: 77–82.
6. Pearce DJ, Spencer L, Hu J et al. Class I topical corticosteroid use by psoriasis patients in an academic practice. J Dermalog Treat 2004; 15: 235–8.
7. Lebwohl M, Freeman AK, Chapman MS et al. Tacrolimus ointment is effective for facial intertriginous psoriasis. J Am Acad Dermatol 2004; 51: 723–30.

Eczematous disorders of facial skin

Eczema of facial skin does not differ fundamentally from eczema anywhere else on the body and with the exception of venous eczema all types of eczema may occur on the face. However, it is true that some types of eczema occur more frequently on facial skin than elsewhere on the body surface and it is also the case that eczema on the face may behave differently compared to the same type of eczema at other body sites. Table 6.1 lists the different types of facial eczema and their relative frequencies.

Eczema of facial skin is generally not difficult to identify as such but it may be more difficult to pinpoint the exact type of eczema present. The itchiness, the diffuse pinkness and scaling and the exudation with or without crusting all suggest that the condition is eczematous in origin. Spongiosis and vesicle formation are important histological features of acute allergic contact dermatitis or photodermatitis but are muted in most other types of facial eczema. Epidermal thickening and parakeratosis may develop in longstanding facial eczema but as lichen simplex chronicus is uncommon on facial skin these features are less prominent at this site.

TABLE 6.1 Types and frequencies of facial eczema

ECZEMA	RELATIVE FREQUENCY	AGE SPECIFICITY
Atopic dermatitis	Very common	Mostly infants, childhood and in young adults Uncommon in elderly
Seborrheic dermatitis	Very common	All ages
Allergic contact dermatitis	Common	Adults
Irritant contact dermatitis	Uncommon	Mostly adults apart from lip-licking cheilitis in childhood
Lichen simplex chronicus	Rare on face	Mid-life and elderly subjects
Pityriasis simplex	Very common	Infants and children

Differential diagnosis of facial eczema

Uncommonly other red and scaling conditions may occur on the face and be difficult to tell apart from eczema. In particular, psoriasis on the face may be difficult to distinguish from seborrheic eczema (syn. dermatitis) – they both cause redness and scaling in patches on the scalp and at the scalp margin as well as in the folds of the external ears and the nasolabial folds. In fact it can be so difficult at times to differentiate the two disorders that some clinicians when confronted with this type of patient do not bother to try and call the condition 'seborrhiasis'. Superficially apposite as the term is, it suggests that there are patients with a genuine 'overlap disorder' when there really is no evidence that this is the case. A more plausible explanation is that when facial seborrheic dermatitis occurs in someone with psoriasis, the latter is precipitated at the dermatitic sites.

Other red scaling itchy disorders occurring on the face that can be confused with eczema include ringworm in which lesions develop not infrequently on facial skin (tinea faciei) – especially in children who cuddle cats and dogs. When the rash is localized and there is a tendency to clear centrally, strenuous efforts are needed to try to identify fungal mycelium microscopically in the superficial scale and by culture. Discoid lupus erythematosus (DLE) also usually occurs in well-defined patches but is persistent and causes dyspigmentation and scarring. It is described in greater detail with the other autoimmune diseases affecting the face in Chapter 8. Ulerythema ophryogenes is a strange persistent scaling disorder of children that often resembles persistent seborrhoeic dermatitis. Solar keratoses, Bowen's disease, superficial basal cell carcinoma and lymphomatous disorders are covered in Chapter 7. Exposure to the sun produces many disorders – some of which are dermatitic and described in this chapter.

Although for the most part all these disorders have their own distinctive clinical appearances, distribution and history, if doubt remains the diagnosis can be settled by the simple expedient of taking a 3 or 4 mm punch biopsy.

Atopic dermatitis

This disorder seems to single out the face for special punishment. Not only is the face the most severely affected site in many patients, it is virtually the only affected site in some. In early infancy there is often symmetrical pinkness and fine scaling of the cheeks and forehead which episodically becomes infected and develops exudation and crusting. In childhood, the cheeks are quite pale, there is periocular darkening and together with the dry, slightly scaling skin surface there is a quite characteristic facial appearance. The most typical clinical changes in atopic dermatitis are seen around the eyes and together with the pallor and dryness mentioned above give rise to a characteristic set of features known as atopic facies (Figure 6.1). The periocular skin is often darker than normal and there is usually a crease beneath the eyes known as the Denny Morgan fold (Figure 6.2). In addition, the eyebrows are sparse and sometimes there are fewer eyelashes than normal. There has been some debate as to whether the Denny Morgan fold is an

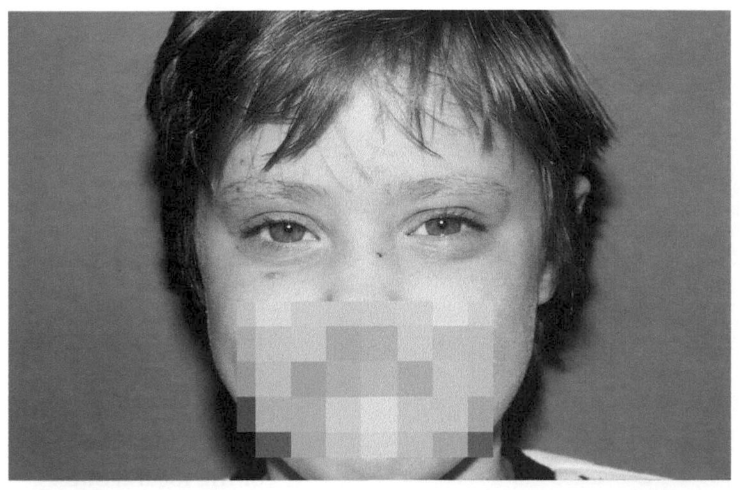

Figure 6.1

Atopic facies. There is reddening around the eyes but some pallor of the cheeks as well as scaling.

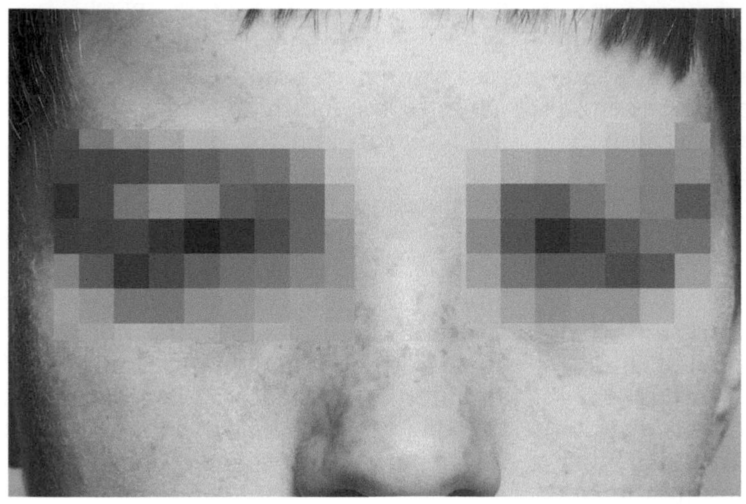

Figure 6.2

There is a fold of skin beneath each eye characteristic of atopic dermatitis. This is known as the Denny Morgan fold.

independent 'marker' of the disease or merely the result of it. Hywel Williams[1] believes it is caused by the eczematization and is not an independent feature. The persistent rubbing of the eyes and surrounding skin to alleviate the irritation is probably the major cause of the various periocular changes. Virtually all atopic dermatitis sufferers use the knuckles of the proximal interphalangeal joints of the index fingers of both hands to rub their eyes and this must result in not inconsiderable damage to the skin and produce a type of lichenification (Figure 6.3). Damage to the eyes themselves can also result from the rubbing, causing the vision-threatening condition of keratomalacia and keratoconus in which softening of the cornea results in altered geometry of this structure and even perforation. Cataracts in subjects with atopic dermatitis

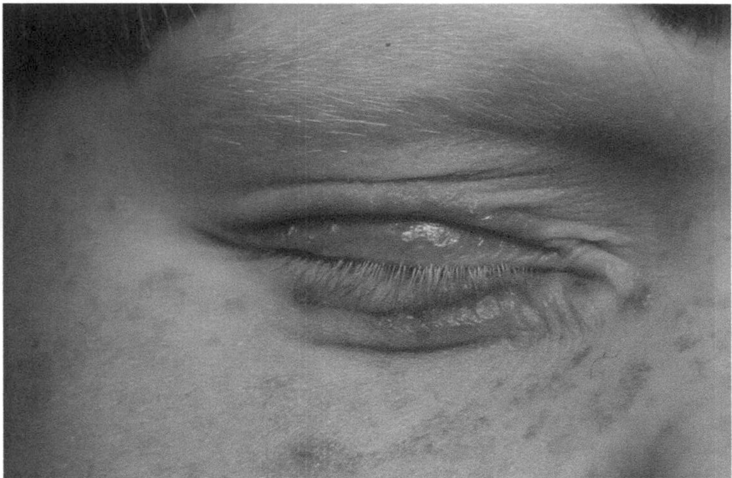

Figure 6.3

Rubbing and scratching of the peri-ocular areas is common in atopic dermatitis, leading to redness and swelling of the local tissues.

occasionally develop but are uncommon and mostly occur in patients with severe and longstanding disease.[2] In some cases it has been suggested that the use of topical steroids may be the cause.[3] It seems unlikely that the rubbing is a causative factor.

Differential diagnosis

When patients give a clear history that their facial rash is precipitated and/or aggravated by exposure to sunlight they may have either actinic prurigo or polymorphic light eruption or some other type of photo dermatitis despite the fact that the condition looks very much like atopic dermatitis. Actinic prurigo (also called Hutchinson's summer prurigo) (see Chapter 7) predominantly affects children aged 8–14 and is virtually restricted to the face (Figure 6.4). This disorder is very itchy and for the most part causes lesions on the nose, cheeks and forehead. Actinic prurigo is precipitated and aggravated by long-wave UVR specifically.

Polymorphic light eruption (PLE) is pre-eminently a disorder of young and middle-aged women. It occurs on all light-exposed skin sites, but mostly the dorsal aspects of the forearms and the neck are affected. The face is less often involved in PLE perhaps because frequent exposure leads to tolerance – in fact this is the basis of treatment with PUVA. Although the condition can look very much like atopic dermatitis, the lesions are not infrequently thicker and more 'prurigo-like' and more heterogeneous. This disorder is also due to exposure to the longer UVR wavelengths of the solar spectrum (UVA).

Two other eczematous conditions need to be distinguished from atopic dermatitis. The first of these is allergic contact dermatitis. The appearance of eczematous lesions at other sites of contact such as on the hands and fingers or the scalp should help distinguish this disorder from atopic dermatitis (see below). The other occasionally confusing condition is not yet dignified by a specific name and is anyway often confused with allergic

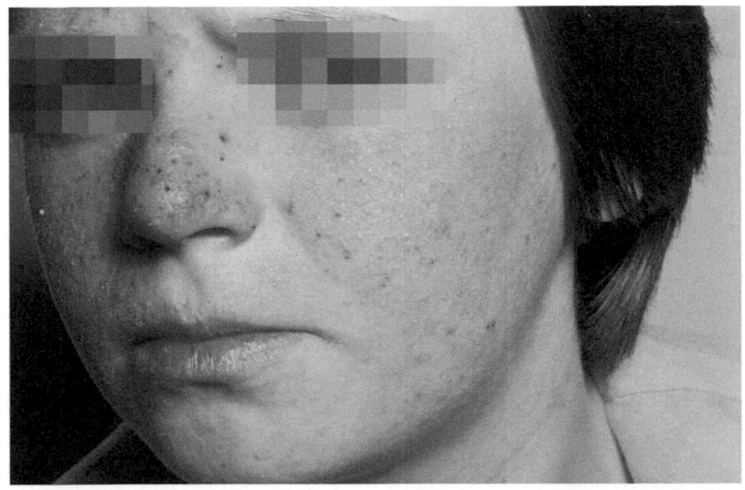

Figure 6.4

This 13-year-old girl has an itchy eczema-like rash on her face in the light-exposed areas typical of actinic prurigo.

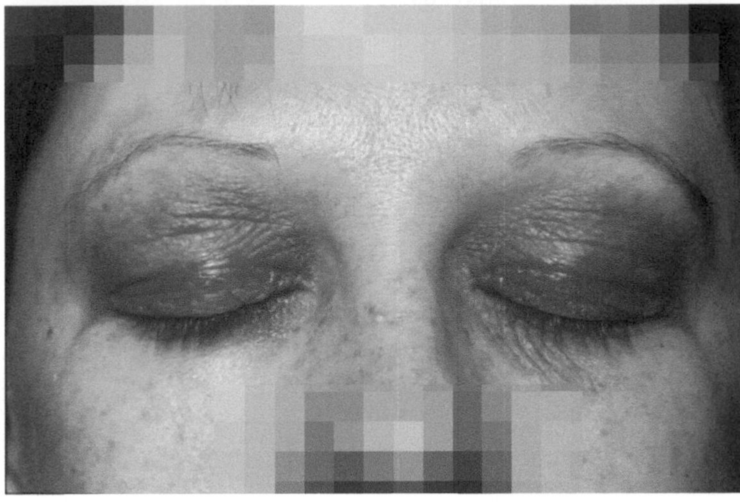

Figure 6.5

This young woman's dermatitis is confined to the eyelids. It is symmetrical and a cause has not been identified.

contact dermatitis. It is eyelid dermatitis in young to middle-aged women. It is symmetrical and restricted to the upper eyelids and to a lesser extent the surrounding periocular skin (Figure 6.5). Typically the women affected complain bitterly of the pruritus as well as the appearance of the condition and, despite every best effort at uncovering a cause, the condition resists all attempts at full characterization and persists stubbornly despite thoughtful and intensive treatment. In most instances of this curious disorder the condition grumbles on for several years.

Cause

The cause and pathogenesis of atopic dermatitis is not completely understood.

Current views suggest that there is an imbalance between different types of T-lymphocytes of the helper type so that there is a comparative deficiency of some cytokines including gamma-interferon and an excess of others such as IL-4. There seems to be a genetic susceptibility to atopic disease[4] but how this fits in with the well-known increased levels of circulating immunoglobulin IgE,[5] the deficiencies of the stratum corneum barrier[6] and the disordered T-cell physiology remains mysterious. Current views are well summarized in reference 7.

Treatment

Patients with atopic dermatitis typically have dry skin all over the entire skin surface and this background xeroderma needs to be managed with frequent applications of emollients acceptable to the patient, the use of moisturizing cleansers and the use of bath oils. The presence of skin infection should be suspected and if found treated with suitable antimicrobial drugs. The principles of treatment for generalized atopic dermatitis are set out in reference 7. The only specific issue with regard to atopic dermatitis as far as the face is concerned is the use of topical corticosteroids. The least potent agent necessary to control the symptoms is the one that should be used. Often moderately potent corticosteroid preparations such as 0.1% betamethasone-17-valerate, are needed and this causes anxiety in patient or parents or both as well as the medical attendant concerning skin atrophy and systemic absorption. The writer is well aware of the hazards of the use of topical corticosteroids on the face, but believes that the problems are not often put into reasonable perspective. The relief from the intense and disabling pruritus obtained with corticosteroid preparations is noticeable in a few days so that prolonged usage may anyway not be required. If the very potent topical corticosteroids such as clobetasol-17-propionate and halcinonide are avoided and the moderately potent agents are not used for more than 2 weeks, it is very unlikely that significant skin thinning or clinically significant systemic absorption will occur.

Topical tacrolimus (0.03%), (Protopic) and pimecrolimus (1.0%) (Elidel) are calcineurin inhibitors and are important new effective alternatives to the topical steroids.

Allergic contact dermatitis

The face is a prime target for allergic contact dermatitis. Allergens may come into contact with the facial skin by direct contact with, for example, a plant or flower, an article of clothing, any agent encountered by the skin of the hands or fingers, or after application of a cosmetic, or fragrance or the use of a medicament. Allergens may be transferred inadvertently via the hands or less frequently be airborne. Some allergens only sensitize in the presence of sunlight and the resulting disorders are known as photodermatoses and are described on page 91. Allergic contact dermatitis possesses the clinical features of any eczematous disorder, but its acuity and distribution over the face are often quite characteristic of the allergen responsible. These characteristic features when combined with a painstakingly careful analysis of the patient's occupation, hobbies and activities, will usually reveal the cause of the problem.

It is nonetheless vital that, regardless of a strong clinical suspicion, formal patch testing is performed to confirm the clinical impression. The results – positive or negative – are of major importance to the final diagnosis and management and justify the minor inconvenience of the procedure. The technique of occlusive patch testing is not learnt overnight and requires attention to detail and considerable experience before reliable results are obtained.[8] Assuming that a suitable patch test system is accessible, what are the most appropriate allergens to use in someone with a facial dermatitis? The European standard battery of 24 allergens together with the battery of common allergens in cosmetics will detect some 90–95% of the allergens responsible for allergic contact dermatitis affecting the face.

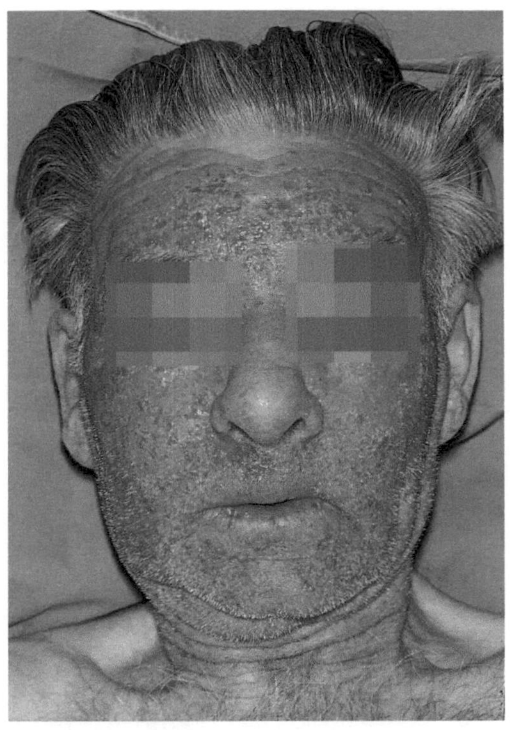

Figure 6.6

Acute allergic contact dermatitis (due to lanolin in a topical preparation).

To illustrate some of the clinical features, a few examples of facial allergic contact dermatitis are given below. Sensitivity to a constituent of a topical preparation can be difficult to sort out as reactions may also occur after use of pharmaceutical preparations used to treat the patient's presenting disorder. Lanolin was at one time a frequent cause of allergic contact dermatitis of the face but is now a much less-frequent problem despite popular belief to the contrary. This is because of the present-day use of preparations from which the plain wool fat has been removed or substituted with a much less allergenic derivative of lanolin. When lanolin sensitivity does occur it produces a generalized facial dermatitis worse in the facial flexures and around the eyes (Figure 6.6). It is also present on the hand that applies the offending topical preparation to the face.

Similar rashes may occur in individuals who develop a sensitivity to other common constituents of topical preparations such as antimicrobial preservatives and fragrances. Neomycin is a well-known sensitizer found in topical preparations which can cause allergic contact dermatitis around the eyes and nose in particular – both sites at which neomycin-containing preparations are often applied (Figure 6.7).

A classic amongst airborne allergens is phosphorus sesquisulphide – liberated

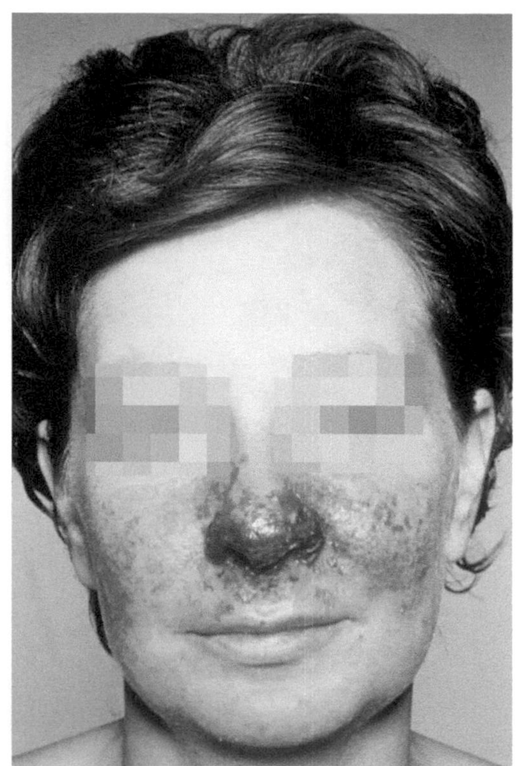

Figure 6.7

Allergic contact dermatitis to neomycin in a topical preparation.

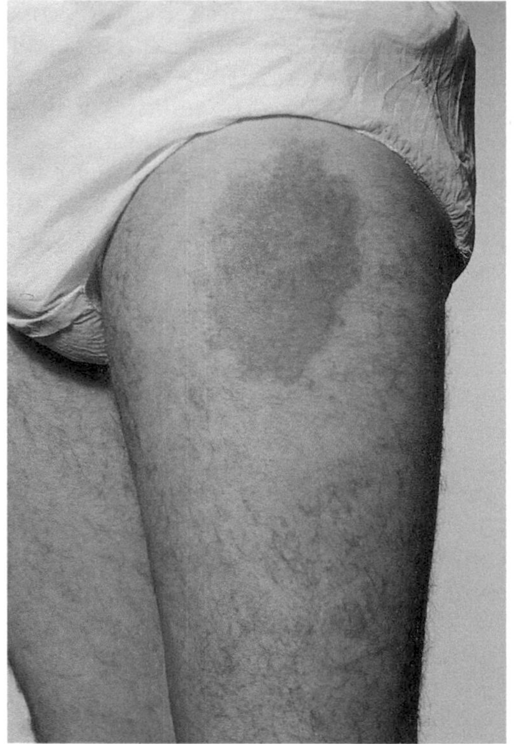

Figure 6.8

Allergic contact dermatitis to phosphorus sesquisulphide from red-headed matches. The patch on the thigh is due to the allergen leaching out of the trouser pocket.

into the puff of smoke that forms when a 'red-headed' match is struck against the strike pad on the side of the match box. Typically pipe smokers are affected at two sites – the upper part of the face (the periocular region in particular) and the lateral aspect of the upper thigh (Figure 6.8). The explanation for the latter site is that the box of matches is usually carried in the trouser pocket, allowing the particles of phosphorus sesquisulphide formed when the match ignites and which stay on the strike pad surface to leach out, contact and ultimately sensitize the skin in contact with the trouser pocket.

Contact with flowers such as those of the Primula family can certainly also cause an acute allergic contact dermatitis. In some unfortunate subjects there is such a high degree of sensitivity that when they enter a room in which there is the particular flower the sensitized individuals almost immediately experience itchiness of exposed sites and within a few hours acute eczema develops with swelling and vesiculation appearing on the face, neck and hands. Chrysanthemums can also cause this type of acute eczematous problem. The Compositae group of plants and some fruits can also cause a photodermatitis affecting the face.

Seborrheic dermatitis

Seborrheic dermatitis is common at all ages and in both sexes. It is by no means confined to facial skin but the face, scalp and neck are frequently affected, although the disease may occur in the absence of facial involvement. On the face it is the flexures that bear the brunt of the disorder although the scalp is often conspicuously involved as well. The rash itself is usually red and scaly (Figures 6.9a and 6.9b) as is eczema elsewhere, but in addition, a few papules and pustules may develop in some patients. On the scalp, dandruff is the predominant physical sign, although in many cases careful inspection of the scalp will also reveal an erythematous

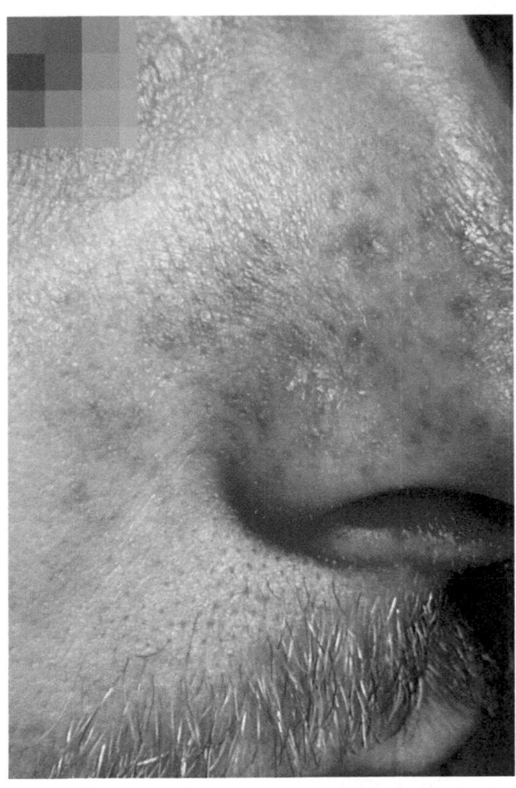

Figure 6.9a

Paranasal seborrheic dermatitis.

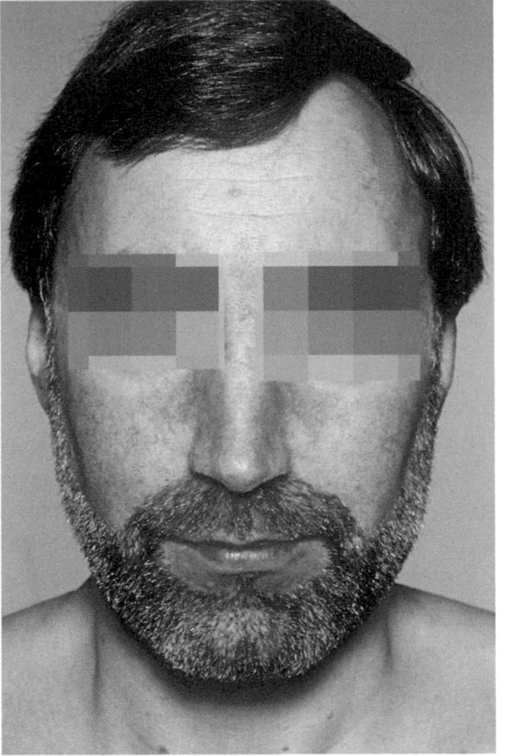

Figure 6.9b

Symmetrical paranasal seborrheic dermatitis.

background. In severely affected patients, exudation and crusting occurs as well as redness and scaling in patches on the scalp and in the facial flexures.

A condition sometimes known as infectious eczematoid dermatitis seems to be related to seborrheic dermatitis. It occurs in acute attacks and mostly affects the middle aged and overweight. On the head and neck it is the ears and the areas around them that are the most dramatically affected.

Patients who have AIDS or who are immunosuppressed for another reason seem particularly susceptible to seborrheic dermatitis. Figure 6.10 illustrates a patient with AIDS who developed seborrheic dermatitis rash following transfusions of HIV-contaminated factor VIII concentrates for hemophilia several years previously and Figure 6.11 shows a woman who had a transient comparative deficiency of T-helper lymphocytes for unknown reasons.[9]

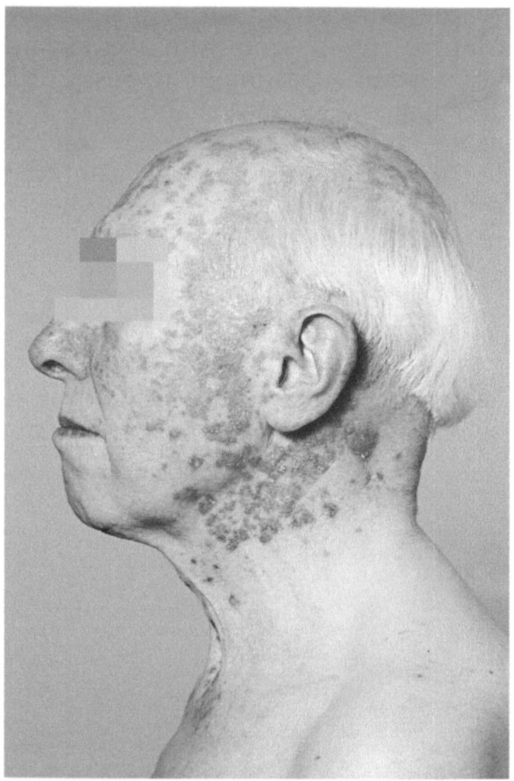

Figure 6.10

Seborrheic dermatitis in patient who had AIDS as a result of infusion of factor viii concentrates for hemophilia.

Cause

The occurrence of seborrheic dermatitis in patients whose immunological defenses are compromised and the response of this disorder to antifungal drugs both support the concept that the disorder is in large part due to the overgrowth and perhaps the metabolic activities of the commensal yeast micro-organism *Pityrosporum ovale.*[10,11] It is uncertain whether all individuals are equally susceptible or how the micro-organisms actually cause the dermatitis or whether other micro-organisms can also produce the clinical picture of seborrheic dermatitis.

Treatment

Most patients with seborrheic dermatitis respond to topical preparations containing an antifungal agent combined with a weak corticosteroid. Preparations containing miconazole, clotrimazole, econazole or ketoconazole combined with hydrocortisone 1% used once or twice daily usually suffice to dampen the fires of seborrheic dermatitis. An alternative is a topical preparation containing 8% lithium succinate, although the mode of action

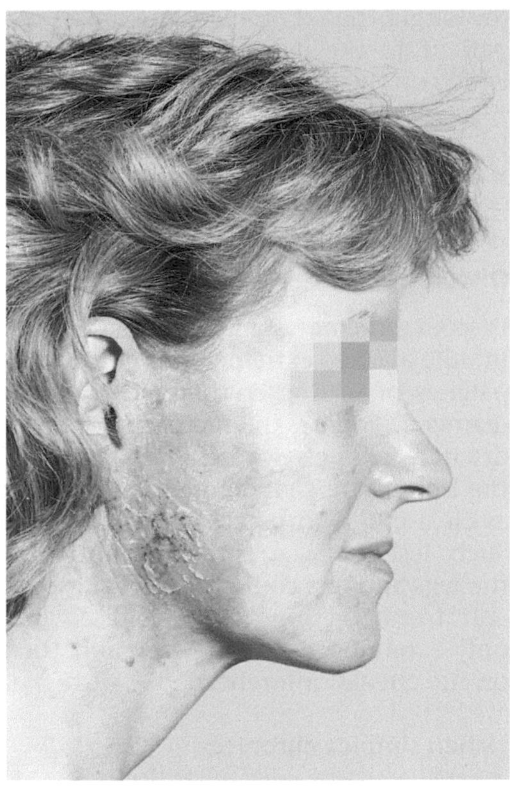

Figure 6.11

This young woman had recalcitrant seborrheic dermatitis and was found to have a deficiency of T-helper lymphocytes.

of this agent is quite uncertain.[12] Older topical preparations containing 2% sulfur with or without salicylic acid are also useful at times for patients with recalcitrant disease. Shampoos containing imidazoles or other antifungal agents such as ketoconazole should also be employed. Tar-containing shampoo preparations were often used and seemed to be moderately active but have fallen under a cloud at the time of writing because of their content of potentially hazardous carcinogenic agents. When investigated, an excess cancer incidence has not been found in users of tar-containing preparations but even a theoretical hazard is undesirable,[13] especially when there are so many non-hazardous alternatives.

Topical tacrolimus (0.1%)[14] and oral terbinafine[15] have also been found helpful in patients with seborrheic dermatitis.

Pityriasis simplex

This odd dermatosis is not uncommon and many patients with it are never brought to the physician's attention as the disorder causes very little in the way of symptoms and only barely perceptible clinical signs. Typically, the disorder occurs in children aged between 2 and 12 years. Pale, somewhat depigmented, discoid patches occur on the cheeks, or sometimes chin, the sides of the neck and maybe the lateral aspects of the upper arms (Figure 6.12). The affected patches develop a fine scaling over the surface and a characteristic whitish appearance and are not usually difficult to diagnose clinically. The hypopigmentation sometimes gives rise to concern in the parents over the possibility of leprosy. Vitiligo and pityriasis versicolor are other possible differential diagnoses. The affected areas tend to resist every best effort at treatment and may last several months. Happily, affected patches eventually resolve and in so doing gradually re-pigment leaving no trace. They may be troublesome in children with black skin as the paler scaling patches are certainly quite noticeable. It has been suggested that the disorder is caused by some sort

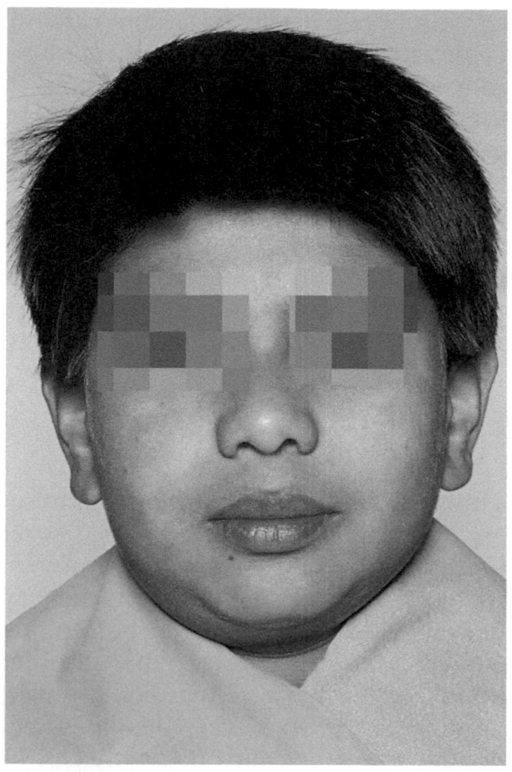

Figure 6.12

Pityriasis simplex is characterized by pale slightly scaling patches on cheeks and chin.

of bacterial infection, but there really is no cultural or microscopic evidence to support this.

Treatment

Combinations of hydrocortisone with an antibacterial agent should be tried (e.g. miconazole and hydrocortisone), together with emollients. Stronger topical corticosteroids may be tried for short periods, but in general the condition is resistant to treatment measures and use for longer than 3 or 4 weeks exposes the patient to the dangers of skin atrophy which on the face is not readily reversible.

Uncommon types of facial eczema

Discoid eczema

Discoid eczema is mainly seen in the middle aged as extremely itchy rounded patches of scaling erythema 2–4 cm in diameter. There is often a background of dry itchy skin elsewhere. The margins of the lesions are well-defined, but are not as clear-cut as in psoriasis or ringworm. Such lesions occur predominantly on the legs and less commonly on the arms and trunk. Lesions of discoid eczema only rarely occur on the face and then on the cheeks or forehead.

Lichen simplex chronicus

This often stress-related aggravatingly itchy disorder is characterized by well-defined, red, scaling (sometimes psoriasiform) and lichenified plaques. It commonly develops on certain sites with great regularity including the ankles, the knees, the wrists, the back of the neck and the occipital region of the scalp. Lichen simplex is quite uncommon on the face, although, as mentioned previously in atopic dermatitis, a form of lichenification occurs round the eyes. It is distressingly quite resistant to treatment.

Irritant contact dermatitis

Dermatitis on the face due to contact with toxic chemicals is not uncommon and is mostly due to transfer of solvents, detergents or other irritants to the face from the hands. All types of eczema can be aggravated by irritating substances in cosmetics or even topical pharmaceutical preparations. When irritant dermatitis does develop on the face the periorbital zones and the neck are the most vulnerable sites and are the first areas to react. Paradoxically, some topical corticosteroids can be quite irritant, particularly cream, gel and lotion preparations because of the emulsifying agents or microbiocides they contain.

Individuals with sensitive skin are prone to irritation from topical acne preparations containing benzoyl peroxide, tretinoin or isotretinoin and tazarotene. This is not uncommon, but is usually of a mild degree and rapidly resolves when the offending preparation is stopped. A mild degree of irritation may also occur with the use of adapalene and azelaic acid preparations. Facial skin irritation may also be a problem with preparations for psoriasis such as those containing calcipotriol, calcitriol, dithranol or tazarotene. Treatment of irritant dermatitis centers round identification of the cause and removal of it. Emollients and weak corticosteroids help relieve symptoms.

Photo aggravation

Eczema that is caused by, precipitated by or aggravated by exposure to the sun can be described as photosensitive eczema. The rash of some patients with atopic dermatitis is worsened by sun exposure. This seems curiously reproducible in the individual patient, but is non-specific in the sense that other agencies can also aggravate the condition and that it does not differ in its overall natural history or clinical appearance from 'ordinary atopic dermatitis'. This and other clinical states in which pre-existing eczema is aggravated by solar exposure will not be further described here. Those disorders in which solar radiation plays a major causative role are usually divided into photo toxic (photo irritant) and photo allergic types.

Photo toxic (photo irritant) dermatitis

This condition mostly presents as an exaggerated sunburn reaction and is due to the causative chemical agent being transformed by elevation to higher energy levels by solar ultraviolet radiation (UVR). It develops a short time after exposure to UVR and unlike photo allergy occurs in a substantial proportion of those exposed. Both agents that are contacted topically and those reaching the skin after systemic administration can be responsible. Examples of substances which cause photo toxic reactions when applied to the skin as therapeutic agents include the psoralens. Such reactions also occur accidentally in phytophotodermatitis. In the latter the psoralens are contained in plant juices and are contacted inadvertently: for example, in bergamot fruit pickers in Southern Europe or by gardeners contacting meadow grass. Tar preparations may also cause photodermatitis.

Photo allergic dermatitis

This form of eczema arises in a few individuals exposed to certain chemical agents and solar ultraviolet radiation of the long-wave type (UVA). It is analogous to allergic contact dermatitis. The eczematous rash starts off by being confined to the light-exposed areas but later the condition may spread to areas that are less obviously exposed. The photo allergen

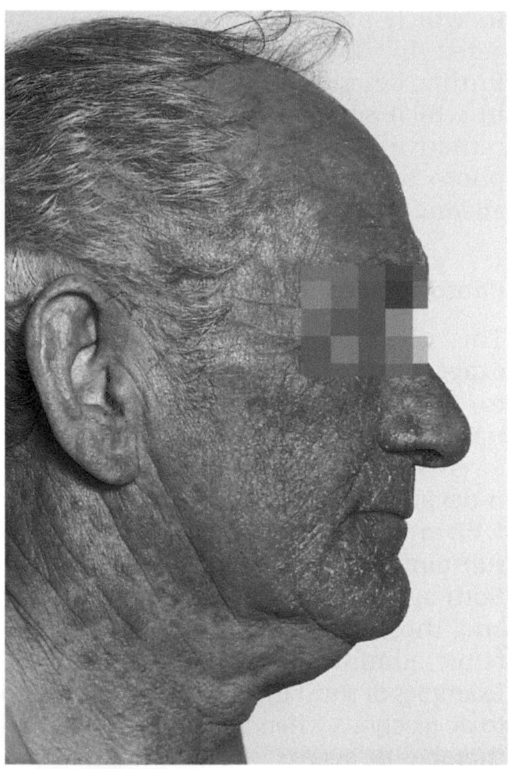

Figure 6.13

This man has chronic actinic dermatitis. The rash is worse on the face but not confined to the exposed areas.

may be contacted topically or, less frequently, reaches the skin by the systemic route. Chemical agents that act as photo allergens include fragrances (e.g. musk ambrette, methyl coumarin), sunscreen constituents (e.g. benzophenone-3, PABA esters) and halogenated salicylanilides (e.g. bithionol, hexachlorophane). Phenothiazines, sulfonamides and griseofulvin are some of the agents that may occasionally cause photo allergic contact dermatitis via the systemic route. The diagnosis is confirmed by photo patch tests in which two sets of patches containing suspected allergens are placed on the skin under occlusion. One set is uncovered after 24 hours and irradiated by long-wave UVR. The irradiated patches alone react in photo contact dermatitis. Treatment must include observation after removal of the identified allergen and protection from long-wave UVR. Photo allergic dermatitis (Figure 6.13) sometimes persists and develops into the condition of chronic actinic dermatitis (see Chapter 7).

References

1. Charman CR, Venn AJ, Williams H. Measuring atopic exzema severity visually: which variables are most important to patients? Arch Dermatol 2005; 141: 1146–51.
2. Nagaki Y, Hayasaka S, Kadoi C. Cataract progression in patients with atopic dermatitis. J Cataract Refract Surg 1999; 25: 96–9.
3. Castrow FF 2nd. Atopic cataracts versus steroid cataracts. J Am Acad Dermatol 1981; 5: 64–6.
4. Cookson WO, Moffatt MF. The genetics of atopic dermatitis. Curr Opin Allergy Clin Immunol 2002; 2: 383.
5. Perkin MR, Strachan DP, Williams HC et al. Natural history of atopic dermatitis and its relationship to serum immunoglobulin E in a population-based birth cohort study. Pediatr Allergy Immunol 2004; 15: 221–9.
6. Hata M, Tokura Y, Takigawa M et al. Assessment of epidermal barrier function by photoacoustic spectrometry in relation to its importance in the pathogenesis of atopic dermatitis. Lab Invest 2002; 82: 1451–61.
7. Taieb A, Hanifin J, Cooper K et al. Proceedings of the 4th Georg Rajka International Symposium on Atopic Dermatitis, Arachon, France, September 15–17, 2005. J Allergy Clin Immunol 2006; 117: 378–90.
8. Albert MR, Gonzalez S, Gonzolez E. Patch testing to a standard series in 608 patients

tested from 1990 to 1997 at Massachusetts General Hospital. Am J Contact Dermat 1998; 9: 207–11.

9. Kurwa HA, Marks R. Protracted cutaneous disorders in association with low $CD4^+$ lymphocyte counts. Br J Dermatol 1995; 133: 625–9.
10. Shuster S. The aetiology of dandruff and the action of therapeutic agents. Br J Dermatol 1984; 111: 235–42.
11. Hay RJ, Graham-Brown RAC. Dandruff and seborrhoeic dermatitis: causes and management. Clin Exp Dermatol 1997; 22: 3–6.
12. Langtry JA, Rowland Payne CM et al. Topical lithium succinate ointment (Efalith) in the treatment of AIDS-related seborrhoeic dermatitis. Clin Exp Dermatol 1997; 22: 216–19.
13. Fijsh JM, Andres LS, Pohl LR et al. Differing degrees of coal tar shampoo induced mutagenesis in the salmonella/liver system in vitro. Pharmacology 1980; 20: 1–8.
14. Braza TJ, Dicarlo JB, Soon SL et al. Tacrolimus (0.1%) ointment for seborrhoeic dermatitis: an open label pilot study. Br J Dermatol 2003; 148: 1242–4.
15. Scaparro E, Quadri G, Virno G et al. Evaluation of the efficacy and tolerability of oral terbinafine (Daskil) in patients with seborrhoeic dermatitis. A multicenter randomized investigator-blinded placebo-controlled trial. Br J Dermatol 2001; 144: 854–7.

Sunlight and facial skin

Facial skin is subjected to daily bombardment by solar radiation and in this chapter I hope to indicate the influence that this has on the health and appearance of this part of the anatomy. I will consider three issues – the nature of the solar stimulus, the susceptibility of the individual and the results of solar exposure.

The solar stimulus

All life on earth is ultimately dependent on the sun as a source of energy so whatever we say about its damaging effects it must be borne in mind that we can't do without it! This flaming incandescent mass some 93 million miles away emits a continuous spectrum of electromagnetic energy which 'bathes' all in its path. Near our planet the solar radiation has to penetrate the atmosphere before it reaches the earth's surface and the skin of individuals who tread its surface. During its journey through the atmosphere segments of the spectrum are absorbed and attenuated dependent on the wavelength and energy of the radiation. The visible light part of the spectrum has very little effect on the biology of the skin. It is the ultraviolet (UV) segments that have the most relevance to us, although the infrared wavelengths at the other end can also affect the skin. The UV radiation (UVR) has wavelengths that span 200–400 nm approximately. It is conventionally divided into short-wave UVR of 200–290 nm (UVC), medium-wave UVR of 290–320 nm (UVB) and long-wave UVR of 320–400 nm (UVA) (Figure 7.1). The atmosphere and in particular the ozone layer (which is equivalent to a layer of 1–2 mm thick) absorbs most of the UVC and a significant proportion of the UVB.

The season of the year, the nearness of the equator and the time of the day determine the path length of the solar UVR to the site on the earth's surface under discussion. It should be evident that the highest dose rate of UVR will be at midday, at the equator, in mid-summer. It is prudent when discussing sun avoidance with patients for one reason or another to advise them to avoid exposure between 11.30 am and 3 pm and to be cautious when outdoors from the end of March to the end of September. Altitude also influences the dose of UVR – the higher one climbs the less protective atmosphere exists above your head and the greater the dose. It is interesting to note that at the Dead Sea in Israel, which is 400 meters below sea level (the lowest point on the earth's surface), much of the sunburning UVB is filtered out by the extra amount of air above the earth's surface.

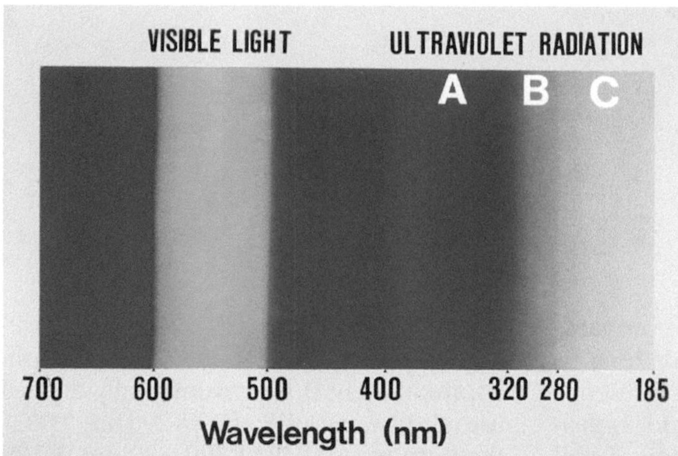

Figure 7.1

Spectrum of visible light and ultraviolet (invisible) radiation from the sun.

Cloud, shade and reflection

Overcast and cloudy skies are not as protective as may be thought. It has been estimated that cloudy gray skies may permit some 70% of the UVR through to the earth's surface – causing nasty unexpected reactions in some who are unaware. Shade is similarly unreliable as a method of protection – trees and fencing often allow sufficient of the sun's rays through to cause a problem.

Reflected UVR can also be damaging. The lighter the color of the surface, the greater the capacity to reflect the sun's rays. The sand, expanses of water, white concrete buildings all reflect efficiently – so that a beach holiday in a Mediterranean or Aegean holiday village can cause serious UVR damage.

Destruction of the ozone layer

The ozone (O_3) is formed by the action of solar UVR on molecular oxygen at the top of the atmosphere. Some of the molecular oxygen splits into atomic oxygen which then unites with the residual unaffected O_2 forming O_3. The ozone is vital to our protection against solar UVR but its function is being threatened by its gradual chemical destruction from a variety of liberated man-made gases. Prominent amongst these are the chlorofluorocarbons (CFCs) – used as propellants in sprays and refrigerants. The destruction of ozone produced by the CFCs is cumulative and long-lasting. The gradual loss of ozone has led to areas of extreme ozone rarefaction or 'holes' through which greatly increased amounts of UVR can reach the earth's surface. It has been estimated that a 1.0% reduction in ozone leads to a 1.2–1.4% increase in carcinogenic effective UVB which could lead to an increase in squamous cell cancer of 2.5% and of basal cell carcinoma of 1.5%.[1] This is potentially extremely serious and has led to international action in an attempt at halting and hopefully reversing this problem.[2]

Susceptibility of the individual and protection against solar damage

It is well known that blonde blue-eyed subjects burn much more easily when exposed to the sun than do darker-skinned types. It is also the case that even with the same degree of skin pigmentation, individuals vary in their sensitivity to the sun. Both of these phenomena need comment. The degree of pigmentation is almost entirely due to the amount of melanin pigment in the skin. This is not a function of the number or size of the melanin-producing cells – the melanocytes. It is, however, a function of the melanin-synthesizing activity of these cells. Melanin absorbs visible light at all wavelengths and UVR and so looks brown-black and protects against UV damage. Melanin is actually two pigments – 'eumelanin', the usual brown-black polymer that accounts for most of the variation in ethnic pigmentation, and 'pheomelanin', a red-brown copper-containing substance which accounts for the reddish skin color of some ethnic types. Individuals with this reddish-brown pigmentation who are also often freckled tend to be very sensitive to the sun and include the Celtic skin types (see later).

In general the darker the degree of skin pigmentation the more protected is the individual against solar damage. Nonetheless even the most heavily pigmented person can be damaged if they are exposed to a sufficiently high dose of UVR (Figure 7.2).

Individuals vary in their sensitivity to the sun independently of their pigmentation and very little is known about the determinants of this variability in the normal population. The variation in sensitivity could have its basis in an as it yet uncharacterized disorder. There are inherited conditions in which mutations cause a deficiency in one of the DNA repair enzymes – the group of disorders known as xeroderma pigmentosum[3] which ultimately result in mutations and skin cancers. Similarly, inherited disorders of porphyrin metabolism result in the deposition of abnormal amounts of photosensitizing porphyrins in the skin and a range of abnormal inflammatory reactions after exposure to the sun.[4] Other clinically well-characterized but as yet metabolically unravelled conditions include Bloom's syndrome and the Rothmund–Thomson syndrome. The 'normal population' varies in its reactivity to chemical irritants and in fact to mechanical stimuli. Similarly it varies in the skin's reactivity to incident UVR. Interestingly, its reactivities

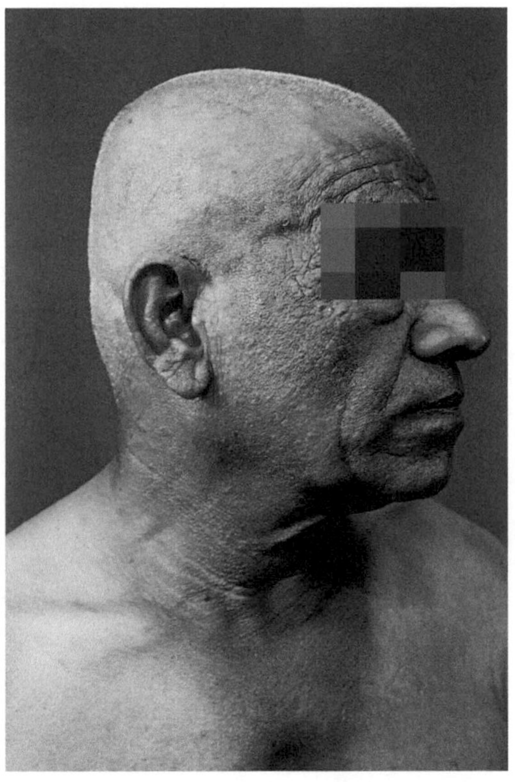

Figure 7.2

This man is an agricultural worker in Sri Lanka. He has quite severe solar damage.

to chemical, mechanical and radiative stimuli seem to be correlated (personal observations) suggesting that the variability resides in some fundamental component of the inflammatory response.

From a practical point of view and regardless of the mechanisms involved it would be useful to have a system categorizing individuals as to their sun sensitivity. Such a system would help in guiding subjects as to the protective measures that they should adopt when exposed to the sun in order to avoid damage. The most often used scheme is known as the Fitzpatrick or Boston classification.[5] This relies on the answers to the questions 'do you burn in the sun?' and 'do you tan after being in the sun?'. The classification is set out in Table 7.1.

Protection against solar damage

Some exposure to the sun is both inevitable and desirable. When considering sun protection it is vital to know the degree of exposure that is expected, where that exposure will occur and of course both the time of the year and time of the day of the exposure. Clearly the advice given will depend on the expected exposure (both time and intensity). It should also depend on the susceptibility of the subject.

Education as to both the short-term and long-term results of sun exposure should form part of the 'protection package' offered, as should information concerning the dangers of relying on shade and the potential usefulness of some items of clothing such as hats (especially when

TABLE 7.1 The Fitzpatrick classification

SKIN TYPE	BURNING	TANNING	MOST OFTEN ASSOCIATED SKIN COLOR
I	Always	Never	Red-haired, freckled skin. Some blondes with blue eyes. Celts
II	Always	Sometimes	Light-brown, hazel or green eyes. Some NW Europeans
III	Sometimes	Always	Brown hair and eyes. Many NW Europeans
IV	Never	Always	Brown-black hair and eyes. Mediterranean types
V	–	–	Asian skin types with brown skin
VI	–	–	African black skin types

there is not much hair!). Some thin garments such as vests, blouses and shirts may actually provide only a small amount of protection, especially if they are made of open-weave materials and it is not particularly unusual to find sunburn beneath such flimsy articles.

It is worthwhile praising the virtues of artificial tans – as at least the amount of sun exposure required to produce the degree of melanization desired is avoided. It is also worthwhile avoiding oils as many enhance the penetration of UVR into the skin.

Sunscreens

Sunscreens are both important and complex and only the briefest of outlines can be given here. The topic is well covered in reference 6. Essentially they are creams, lotions, gels or sprays that are formulated to absorb or reflect solar UVR. They need to be safe to use both as far as the skin to which they are applied is concerned and with regard to the systemic absorption of the compounds that they contain. They protect against UVR but do not protect equally against the different wavelengths. Protection against sunburn (UVB-induced) is measured by the sun protection factor (SPF) and protection against UVA (long-wave UVR) is measured as a protection factor as well. Of value is also the ratio between UVB and UVA protection which is expressed as a number of stars (1–5 stars). The SPF is a very valuable indicator of the degree of protection against UVB as it is a ratio between the time in minutes required for radiated skin protected by the sun screen to develop erythema compared to unprotected skin – thus skin protected by a sunscreen of SPF 20 would have to be irradiated for 20 times longer than unprotected skin before sunburn erythema developed. Apart from sunburn, solar UVB also causes skin cancer, 'photoaging' and depression of delayed hypersensitivity (see below) and sunscreens with high SPF values should also protect against these disorders. However, because it is cumulated UVR damage over long periods that is responsible for these problems it is much less easy to demonstrate this protection experimentally. Nonetheless, there is some evidence that sunscreens do provide these protective qualities as well as protection against sunburn.[7,8]

Long-wave UVR contributes to photocarcinogenesis and is thought to play a major role in 'photoaging'. In addition UVA wavelengths are involved in the photodermatoses (see below), making the use of sunscreens protecting against UVA mandatory in patients with one of these skin disorders. Sunscreens contain substances that either absorb the damaging wavelengths or reflect off the harmful rays. The 'absorbers' are many and various – those that are in common use are set out in Table 7.2. There is an increasingly appreciated problem with these agents in that they become 'activated' when they absorb UVR and then become sensitizers causing a photodermatitis.[9] The reflectants are set out in Table 7.3. The most frequently used reflectant is micronized titanium dioxide. Unfortunately it is quite difficult to get rid of the white 'clown-like' appearance that preparations containing this substance impart to the skin. The other important issue is that the degree of protection offered by the reflectants is not great.

TABLE 7.2	Sunscreen filters (or absorbers)
p-Aminobenzoic acid (PABA; one of oldest sunscreens)	
Diethanolamine *p*-methoxycinnamate (good UVB absorbance)	
2-Ethylhexyl salicylate	
Homomenthyl salicylate	
Glyceryl aminobenzoate	
Triethanolamine salicylate	
Oxybenizone and dioxybenzone	
Sulisobenzone	
Methyl anthranilate	
Octyldimethyl PABA	
Octyl *p*-methoxycinnamate	
Benzophenone–3	
Phenylbenzimidazole sulfonic acid	
Benzylidene camphor sulfonic acid	
Octocrylene	
Ethylhexyl triazone	
Polysilicone–15	
Methylene bis-benzotriazoly1 tetramethy1buty1pheno1	

The above are examples of sunscreen filters.

TABLE 7.3	Sunscreen reflectant agents
Micronized titanium dioxide	
Zinc oxide	
Iron oxide	

Apart from doubts about efficacy in some situations, the biggest problem with the sunscreens has been to get people to use them appropriately and when needed. For this reason sunscreens need to be attractive and pleasant to use. They also need to be 'substantive' to the stratum corneum so that they stick to the skin, don't wash off easily and don't have to be frequently reapplied.

The results of solar exposure

It is not generally appreciated that adult vitamin D deficiency and insufficiency are quite common even in developed European countries. It has been estimated that in the UK vitamin D deficiency occurs in approximately 14.5%[10] of adults and is even higher in the elderly. Sufficient vitamin D is synthesized in the skin by 'exposure of hands, arms, face or back to suberythermal doses of UVR in the UK from April to September for 15 minutes three times per week'.[11] Clearly some sun exposure is important! However, it is not only our vitamin D levels that suffer if we completely shut ourselves off from the sun as some sun exposure is important for our psychological well-being.

Mostly sun exposure causes problems. When exposed to excessive amounts it causes sunburn. The exposure needed to do this depends on all the factors discussed above but even in the comparatively sun-impoverished UK 20 minutes exposure at mid-day in May to August will produce burning on unprotected skin of a type II or type III person. Sunburn is the result of epidermal damage and the liberation of mediators (prostaglandins) and cytokines causing vasodilation and inflammation. Anyone who has had sunburn knows how painful and tender the affected areas are (Figure 7.3). In severely affected patients even blistering can occur. The condition begins 8–16 hours after exposure and lasts 3–5 days – tanning occurring subsequently. This type of acute solar injury is not only the cause of acute discomfort at the time but also seems to increase the risk of melanoma developing in later years.[12] Interestingly children who develop sunburn seem to have a larger number of melanocytic 'nevi' on the sun-exposed sites.[13]

Exposure to UVR depresses cell-mediated immunity.[14] This is partly due to reduction in Langerhans cell numbers and function but also due to an effect on the balance of *cis–trans* isomerization of urocanic acid and on lymphocyte trafficking.

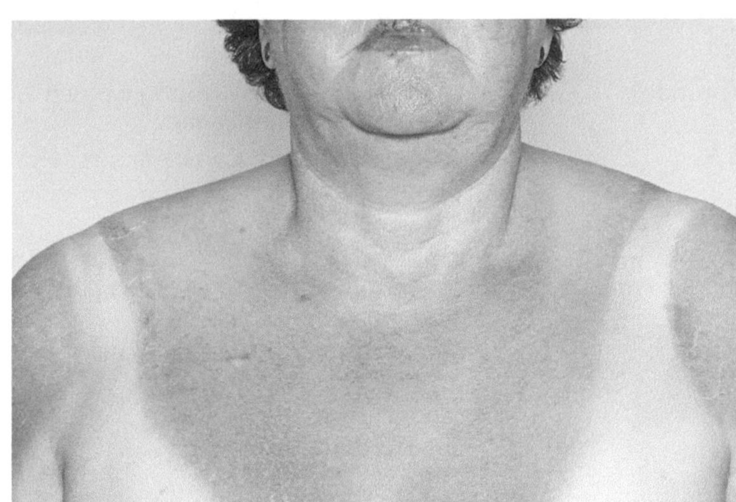

Figure 7.3

Sunburn. Note the sharp 'cut off' between the burnt skin and the protected skin under the 'bra' strap.

The depressed immunity may be part of the mechanism of photocarcinogenesis.

The photodermatoses

The photodermatoses are a group of inflammatory dermatoses which are caused by exposure to solar UVR. Table 7.4 lists the most important of these. In addition to these, there are conditions which seem precipitated and/or aggravated but not actually caused by solar UVR. Discoid lupus erythematosus, for example, is often precipitated by and aggravated by sun exposure. A few patients with atopic dermatitis and some with psoriasis are worsened by being out in the sun. Rosacea is often aggravated by sun exposure

Polymorphic light eruption

This disorder appears to be much more frequent than was once thought – particularly in middle-aged women. Prevalence rates of 15% have been suggested.[15] The rash is mostly papular and/or scaling and

TABLE 7.4 The photodermatoses

DISORDER	COMMENT
Photodermatitis	Due to contact with certain materials
– photoirritant, contact dermatitis (including phytophoto contact dermatitis)	
– photoallergic contact dermatitis	
Polymorphic light eruption	Common, women mainly
Solar urticaria	Uncommon urticarial rash on sun-exposed sites
Actinic prurigo (Hutchinson's summer prurigo)	Itchy dermatitic rash – young women mainly. Cause unknown
Chronic actinic dermatitis	Mainly elderly men. Can be exquisitely sensitive to UVR
Porphyrias	
– erythropoietic pophyria	Recessive. Severely mutilating
– erythropoietic protoporphyria	Dominant. Episodes severe, skin pain and inflammation
– porphyria cutanea tarda	Blistering rash and scleroderma-like change
– variegate porphyria	As above, with episodes as in acute intermittent porphyria

pruritic and develops predominantly on the forearms and neck in the spring and summer (Figure 7.4). Treatment with topical steroids and sunscreens is usually sufficient though severely affected patients can be 'desensitized' by exposure to increasing doses of UVR early in the year before the eruption is due to start.

Solar urticaria

In this quite rare and sometimes disabling condition there is an urticarial response to exposure to particular wavelengths of UVR at the sites of exposure which persists for one or more hours after radiation. Sensitivity is often to a broad band of UVR. It has been established (when such tests were allowed) that the solar sensitivity can be passively transferred in patients' serum when injected intracutaneously into a normal subject – indicating that the agent responsible was in the blood of the affected individual. Desensitization by exposure to increasing doses of the wavelengths responsible can give at least temporary relief.

Actinic prurigo

This dermatosis occurs mostly in young women and resolves in adolescence. Itchy pruriginous papules at exposed sites are characteristic and may resemble atopic dermatitis. It is often familial and is more often seen in Amerindians.

Chronic actinic dermatitis

This not uncommon disorder, which is seen more commonly in middle-aged and elderly men, seems to have become more common in the past 2–3 decades. It has, at various times, been called persistent light reaction photosensitivity eczema, photosensitivity dermatitis and actinic reticuloid. Patients may be exquisitely sensitive to a wide variety of wavelengths, and sensitivity to wavelengths in the UVB, UVA and even visible wavelengths have all been recorded. The rash in some individuals seems to have started with a sensitivity to a halogenated antimicrobial such as tribromosalicyalanilide or bithionol. The areas of skin involved are the

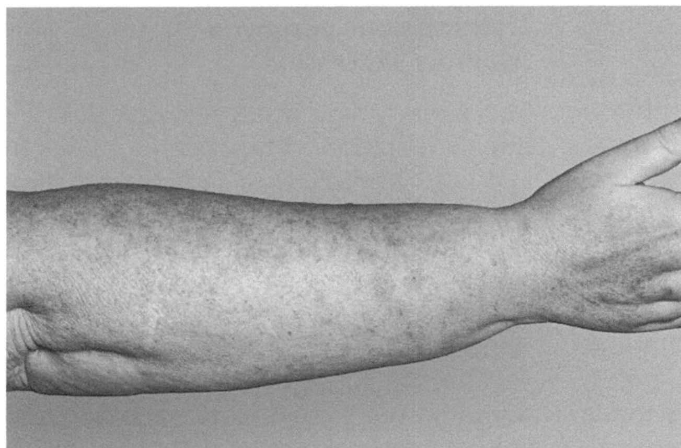

Figure 7.4

Polymorphic light eruption presenting as a maculopapular rash on the forearms.

light-exposed sites at first but later non-exposed skin becomes affected and even the palms are not infrequently involved. The rash is scaling and lichenified and may be quite pigmented. Histologically apart from the eczematous changes there is a variably heavy inflammatory cell infiltrate which when very dense can be quite lymphoma-like. Treatment is by careful sun protection, emollients and topical corticosteroids and if warranted oral azathioprine or ciclosporine. PUVA has also been used under a 'corticosteroid cover'.

The porphyrias

The porphyrias are a group of inherited metabolic disorders in which particular porphyrins collect in abnormal amounts and cause various clinical effects including photosensitivity. The 'hepatic porphyrias' are porphyrias in which liver abnormalities are intimately involved in the metabolic dysfunction. What follows is a very brief description of those porphyrias that show skin lesions. A full description can be found in reference 4.

Porphyria cutanea tarda (PCT)

This disorder is manifested as a photosensitivity and due to a disorder of porphyrin metabolism caused by a deficiency of the enzyme uroporphyrinogen decarboxylase. Characteristically blisters form subepidermally after UVR exposure and heal with scarring and pigmentation. At the affected sites there are, often, apart from the sclerodermiform change and pigmentation, multiple milia and curiously, an excess of terminal hair. The diagnosis is made by finding an excess of coproporphyrins in the urine and stools. This disorder often presents in subjects with pre-existing or concurrent liver disease and is more common in chronic alcoholics. Treatment is directed towards depleting the body's iron stores by repeated venesection (one unit every 1–2 weeks). It may be that the reduced iron improves the activity of the deficient decarboxylase enzyme. Low-dose chloroquine (125 mg twice weekly) also improves PCT by inhibiting porphyrin formation and complexing with uroporphyrin.

Variegate porphyria (VP)

While uncommon in Europe this type of porphyria is much more common in South African citizens of Dutch descent. It is due to a dominantly inherited mutation in protoporphyrinogen oxidase. There is however 'low penetrance' so that 80% of affected individuals are asymptomatic. The skin lesions are clinically indistinguishable from PCT but in addition VP patients are subject to attacks of the more serious acute porphyria with severe abdominal pain and a motor peripheral neuropathy. Avoidance of sun exposure, alcohol and of systemically administered drugs are important components of the management.

Erythropoietic porphyria (Günther's disease)

This is an extremely rare recessive disorder due to deficiency of uroporphyrinogen III synthase leading to a massive overproduction of type I porphyrins. Clinically the blistering and erosions are much more severe than those in PCT and there is considerable destruction, scarring and pigmentation with marked hirsutes completing the horrific disfigurement. There is an accompanying hemolytic anemia and splenomegaly which may be responsible for a thrombocytopenia.

Erythropoietic protoporphyria (EPP)

This is inherited as an autosomal dominant condition although only a small proportion of those affected develop any symptoms. It is the result of a ferrochelatase deficiency resulting in the overproduction of protoporphyrin IX. Onset is usually in childhood with the complaint of 'severe burning pain' and a pricking sensation experienced a few minutes after sun exposure which persists for several hours. The affected skin may show few clinical signs although erythema swelling and erosions develop in some. Patients accumulate protoporphyrin and may develop liver disease.

> Long continued exposure to solar UVR has two other major effects on the skin – the production of skin cancers and the changes known collectively as photoaging.

Non-melanoma skin cancer

There can be no doubt that solar exposure is responsible for most non-melanoma skin cancers and precancer (NMSC) including solar keratoses, Bowen's disease, squamous cell carcinoma and basal cell carcinoma. The evidence for the causative role of UVR is as follows:

- most NMSC occurs on the exposed skin (face, forearms and bald scalp)
- much more NMSC occurs in countries near the equator where the dose of UVR received is much greater
- much more NMSC occurs in light-skinned individuals with little photoprotective melanin
- more NMSC occurs in those who are occupationally exposed to the sun, such as agricultural workers, construction workers and sailors
- there is a high incidence of NMSC in psoriatic patients who have received therapeutic UVR
- NMSC can be induced experimentally by irradiating small mammals with UVR.

The cancers and precancers caused by sun exposure include solar keratoses, intraepidermal epithelioma (Bowen's disease), keratoacanthoma and squamous cell carcinoma. None of these is uniquely due to solar exposure. Interestingly only some 70% of basal cell carcinomas are in light-exposed sites and some appear to arise as the result of developmental anomalies in covered areas.

Increased prevalence

NMSC in all forms have shown a major increase in prevalence and incidence in the past half century. The reasons for this are many and varied but they include greater exposure to the sun because of the decreased working week and increased vacation entitlement. In addition the decreased cost of air travel and package holidays to sunny countries have contributed to the increased annual dose of UVR to the average European citizen. Compounding these social trends there has at the same time grown up the dual ambition to become sun tanned and to live an outdoor 'sporting healthy' lifestyle. The net result of all the socioeconomic alterations is a spiraling increase in skin cancer.[16,17]

Melanoma

Because melanoma is a more lethal disorder than NMSC, records of the increasing incidence of this disorder are both more readily available and more reliable.

The incidence of melanoma has doubled each decade since records began. This increase has been worldwide although the actual numbers are much greater in sunny countries. Even in Glasgow the incidence has increased by approximately 10% per annum since 1971.[18] It has been computed that the average US citizen now has more than a 1 in 75 lifetime risk of developing melanoma.

Curiously melanoma is by no means restricted to the exposed sites of the body and although there is an overall relationship between development of melanoma and cumulated dose of UVR this is not true for the individual skin sites affected. Various possible explanations have been advanced including that sun exposure had been sufficiently suppressive in the past to cell-mediated immunity as to allow neoplastic diseases to develop. It has also been suggested that short sharp episodes of exposure are particularly damaging and that these may not be remembered. A further possibility is that radiation at one site causes the liberation of a 'melanoma factor' which somehow affects other non-exposed areas. None of the above seem particularly convincing and we are left with the 'untidy' observation that melanoma is very much more common in those who have been exposed to large amounts of solar UVR but not at the sun-exposed sites.

Photoaging

The term photoaging is not really satisfactory as it implies that sun exposure is responsible for the changes of aging. In fact sun exposure causes skin damage and because these changes increase with age we associate them with the aging process. Indeed what we see in the exposed skin of the elderly is a combination of cumulated photodamage and intrinsic aging which is inevitable and occurs in all tissues with increasing age. Figure 7.5 demonstrates the changes due to long-continued exposure to the sun on the arm. The skin of the forearms is irregularly pigmented and shows wrinkling

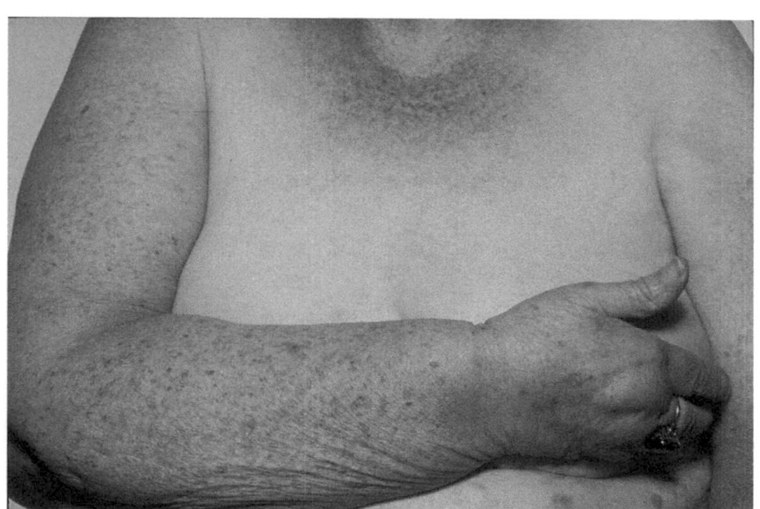

Figure 7.5

This photograph demonstrates solar damage in the exposed skin of the forearm compared to the chest of the same individual giving the impression of aging.

and surface blemishes and irregularities while the non-exposed truncal skin shows no such change although of the same chronological age.

Solar elastosis

Most of the clinical changes observed are due to an alteration in the upper dermis known as solar elastotic degenerative change – or simply solar elastosis. In this, the normal fibrillar collagen is replaced wholly or in part by a morphologically abnormal substance consisting of both a short-stranded 'chopped up' material and deposits of a globular homogeneous material – giving a spaghetti and meat-ball appearance (Figure 7.6). This curious replacement for dermal collagen stains for elastic tissue (Figure 7.7) and all analytical studies have shown that it is in fact a type of elastic tissue[19]. The pathogenesis of this odd elastotic degenerative change in the dermal connective tissue is complex and appears to be due both to the 'upregulation' of elastic tissue synthesis[20] and the activation of metalloproteinases[21] removing the normal upper dermal collagen.

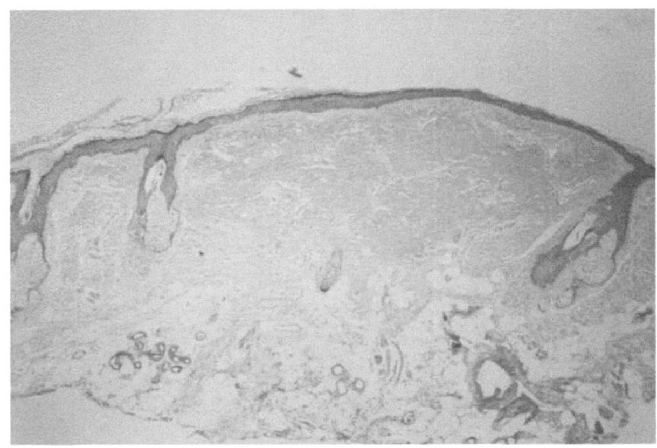

Figure 7.6

Photomicrograph to show solar elastotic degenerative change. There is a slightly basophilic disorganized area of the upper dermis where the normal fibrous nature of the dermis has been lost (hematoxylin and eosin × 30).

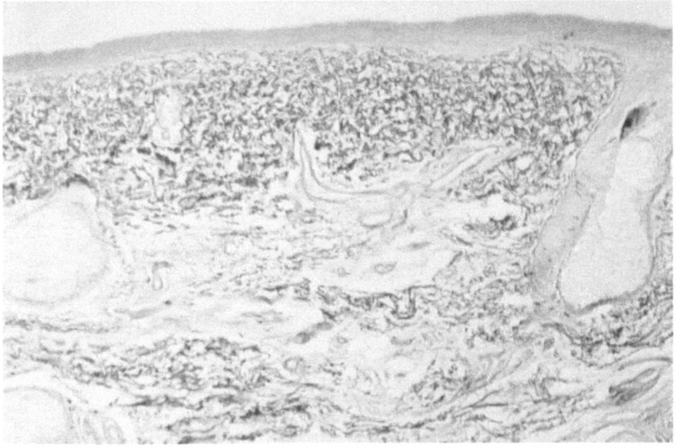

Figure 7.7

Solar elastotic degenerative change. This section has been stained with Halmi's stain to demonstrate elastic tissue. The elastic tissue is demonstrated as a mauve purple area subepidermally (× 45).

Clinical changes due to solar elastosis

The abnormal dermal connective tissue alters both the appearance and the mechanical function of sun-exposed skin. Paradoxically the deposition of abnormal elastic tissue appears to destroy the normal elasticity and the extensibility of the skin so that lines and wrinkles start to appear (Figure 7.8). Furthermore the normal supporting perivascular connective tissue framework is replaced by ineffectual degenerate material allowing the small blood vessels to dilate and become telangiectatic (Figure 7.9). In addition the background color of the skin takes on a pasty dull yellowish hue – known as 'peau citrine'. The pattern of lines and wrinkles depends on the severity of the process, the habitual movement of the face, and the geometry of the face. Lines radiating from the eyes are known as crow's feet and supposedly are due to screwing the eyes up against the sun (Figure 7.10). Short lines radiating from the mouth are associated with cigarette smoking (Figure 7.11) and there is little doubt that smoking does increase the degree of solar elastosis.[22] Deep furrows dividing the back of the neck into a rhomboidal pattern in fair-skinned elderly and middle-aged men is sometimes known as sailors' skin (Figure 7.12) and is associated with serious solar injury to the back of the neck. Photodamaged forearm skin often shows purpuric patches – so-called senile purpura but better termed solar purpura (Figure 7.9a). These purpuric areas are presumably due to injury to dilated and relatively unprotected small superficial blood vessels. The purple patches tend to hang around for several weeks.

Another lesion sometimes evident in photodamaged skin is the triradiate or stellate scar. This irregular scar cannot usually be ascribed to a particular injury and its pathogenesis is uncertain.

Solar keratoses are warty or scaling patches that are the first signs of significant solar damage to the epidermis leading to non-melanoma skin cancer (see page 134). Chronic solar damage is also responsible for senile (solar) lentigines. These are

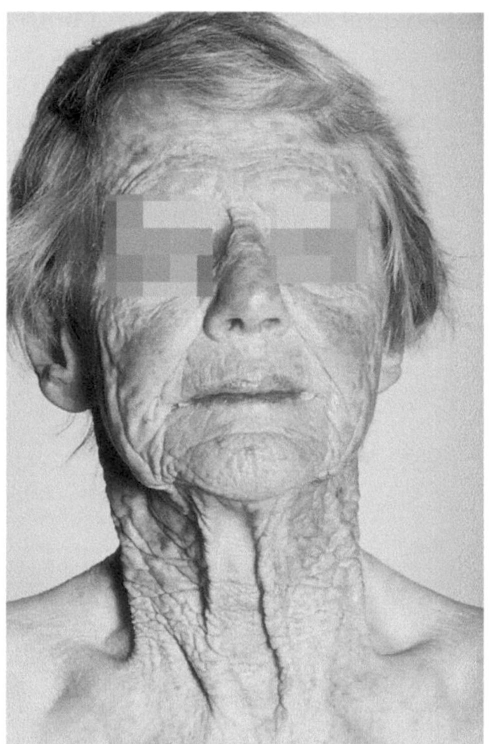

Figure 7.8

This lady shows many lines, wrinkles and furrows – most of which are due to photodamage. Note the yellowish background tinge to the skin (peau citrine).

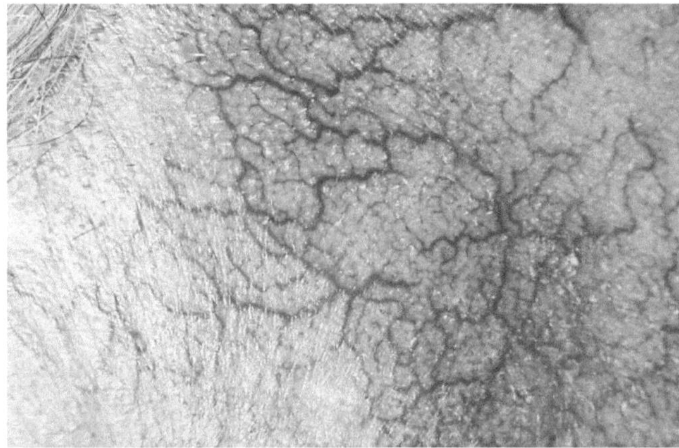

Figure 7.9

Facial telangiectasia of cheek in photodamaged man.

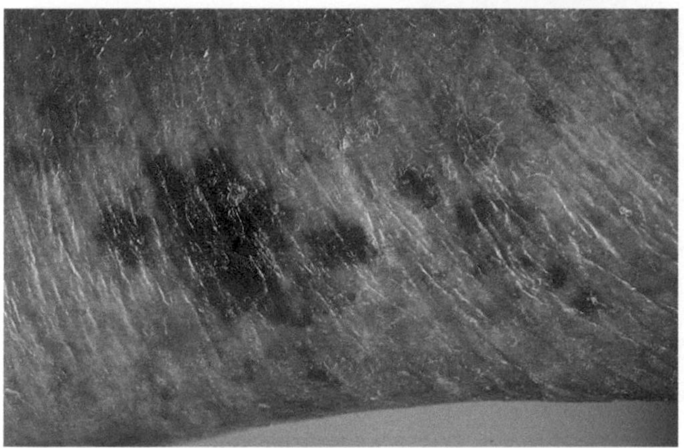

Figure 7.9a

Senile (solar) purpura. This is a frequent accompaniment of photodamage on the forearms.

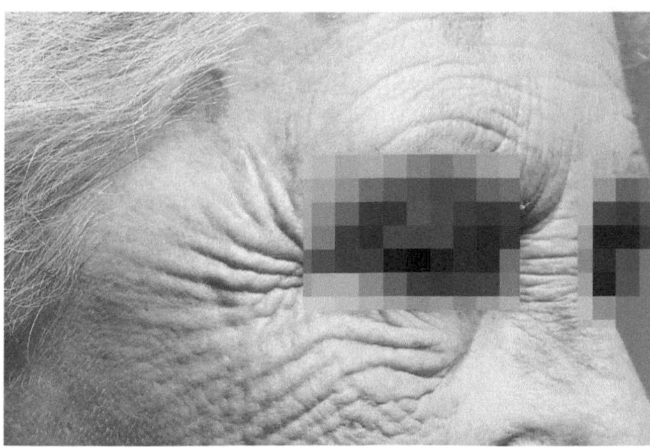

Figure 7.10

'Crowsfeet' – the name given to lines at the corner of the eyes seen in photodamaged subjects.

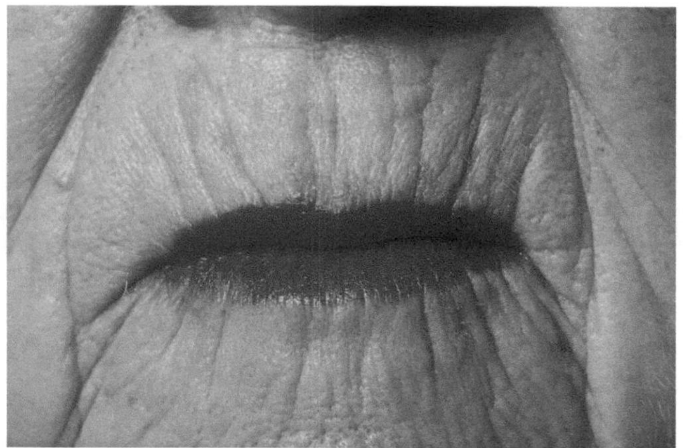

Figure 7.11

The lines around the mouth are due to photodamage although reputedly due to cigarette smoking – the increased elastosis in smokers is not confined to the skin around the mouth.

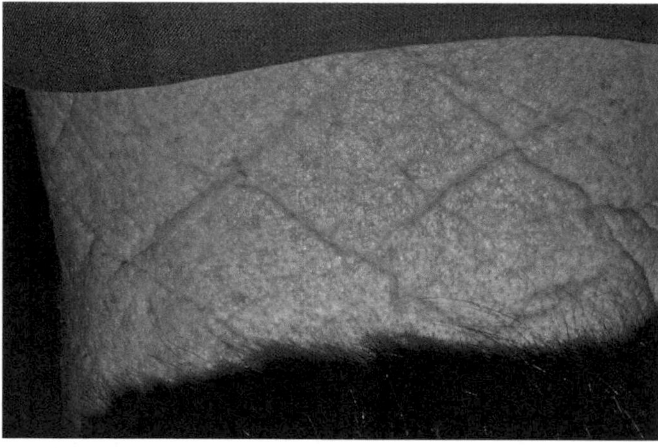

Figure 7.12

Cutis rhomboidalis nuchae (sailors' skin).

irregular flat brown macules occurring on the backs of the hands or the side of the face. Often known as liver spots, they are more often seen in darker-skinned European subjects (Figure 7.13). There is some overlap between these lesions and flat seborrheic warts.

The treatment of chronic photodamage

The use of sunscreens and limitation of sun exposure should both be recommended to prevent further damage. The regular use of emollients gives temporary help in reducing the appearance of lines and wrinkles and by giving an attractive 'bloom' to the skin.

The topical retinoids (tretinoin[23,24], isotretinoin[25] and tazarotene[26]) have all been shown to reduce the signs of solar elastosis. They appear to stimulate the formation of new dermal collagen as well as regularize epidermal and melanocyte structure and function. Clinical improvement starts 3–4 months after use of the

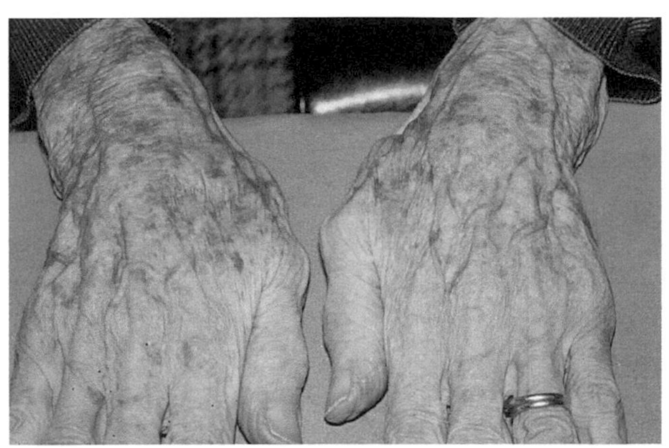

Figure 7.13

The brown macules on the dorsa of the hands are known as senile lentigines but are due to long continued solar exposure.

topical retinoid and increases for the next 6 months before 'plateauing'.[27] Unfortunately these agents do cause irritation and fair-skinned individuals may not be able to tolerate this treatment. Other ways of decreasing the clinical changes of photodamage include laser resurfacing[28] and chemical peeling with 70% glycolic acid or trichloracetic acid – all these agents cause superficial damage to the skin and appear to stimulate new collagen formation.

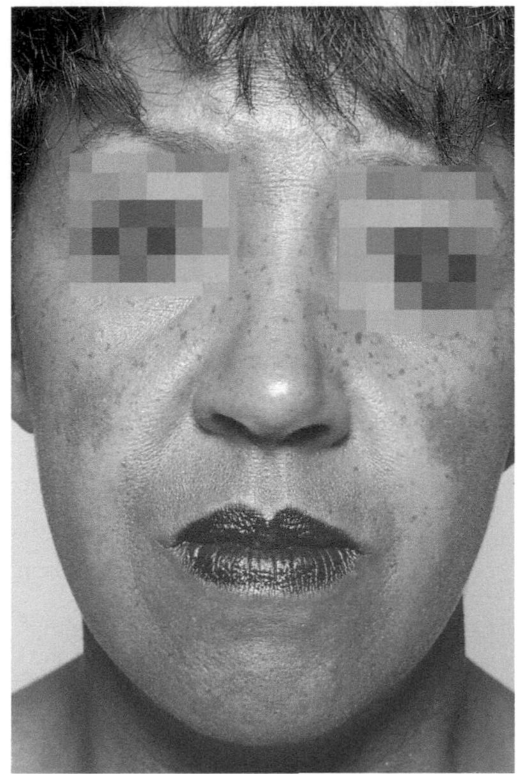

Figure 7.14

The patchy facial pigmentation is known as melasma.

Melasma

Melasma (or chloasma) is a pigmentary disorder affecting the facial skin of women. The pigmentation affects the forehead, cheeks and chin predominantly (Figure 7.14). It often occurs during pregnancy but is by no means restricted to it. It is believed to be related to hormonal status and the oral contraceptive in some patients. It does occur in men but is very uncommon. Treatment is with preparations containing hydroquinnone often with tretinoin as well. Preparations containing azelaic acid (15-20%) are also employed and are quite effective in some patients.

References

1. Diffey BL. Human exposure to ultraviolet radiation. In: Hawk JLM, ed. Photodermatology. London: Arnold, 1999: 5–24.
2. United Nations Environment Programme. Environmental Effects of Ozone Depletion. UNEP 1991: Update.
3. Boulikas T. Xeroderma pigmentosum and molecular cloning of DNA repair genes. Anticancer Res 1996; 16: 693–708.
4. Elder GH. The cutaneous porphyrias. In Hawk JLM, ed. Photodermatology. London: Arnold, 1999: 171–98.
5. Pathak MA, Fitzpatrick TB.Preventative treatment of sunburn dermato-heliosis and skin cancer with sun protective agents. In: Fitzpatrick TB, ed. Dermatology in General Medicine. New York: McGraw Hill, 1993: Vol. 4, 1684.
6. Lowe NJ. Photoprotection. In: Hawk JLM, ed. Photodermatology. London: Arnold, 1999: 213–21.
7. Thompson SC, Jolly D, Marks R. Reduction of solar keratoses by regular sun screen use. N Engl J Med 1993; 329: 1147–51.
8. Boyd AS, Naylor M, Cameron GS et al. The effects of chronic sunscreen use on the histological changes of dermatoheloisis. J Am Acad Dermatol 1995; 33: 941–6.
9. Ferguson J. Drug and chemical photosensitivity. In: Hawk JLM, ed. Photodermatology. London: Arnold, 1999: 155–70.
10. Drugs and Therapeutics Bulletin. Primary vitamin D deficiency in adults. Drug Therap Bull 2006; 44: 25–9.
11. Holick MF. The underappreciated D-lightful hormone that is important for skeletal and cellular health. Curr Opin Endocrinol Diab 2002; 9: 87–98.
12. Oliveria SA, Saraiya M, Geller AC et al. Sun exposure and risk of melanoma. Arch Dis Child 2006; 91: 131–8.
13. English DR, Milne E, Simpson JA. Ultraviolet radiation at places of residence and the development of melanocytic naevi in children (Australia). Cancer Causes Control 2006; 17: 103–7.
14. Ortonne JP, Marks R. The effects of sun exposure on the immune response. In: Photodamaged Skin. London: Martin Dunitz, 1999: 97–107.
15. Pao C, Norris PG, Corbett M et al. Polymorphic light eruption; prevalence in Australia and England. Br J Dermatol 1994; 130: 62–4.
16. Kaufman AJ. The rising incidence of skin cancer in young women. The Skin Cancer Foundation Journal 2006; 24: 17–19.
17. Holme SA, Malinovszky K, Roberts DL. Changing trends non melanoma skin Cancer in South Wales. 1988–98. Br J Dermatol 2000; 143: 1224–9.
18. Mackie RM, Braij CA, Hole DJ et al. Incidence of and survival from malignant melanoma in Scotland: an epidemiological study. Lancet 2002; 360: 587–91.
19. Lovell C, Plastow SR, Russell-Jones R et al. Collagen and elastin in actinic elastosis. J Invest Dermatol 1984; 82: 566.
20. Bernstein EF, Chen YQ, Tamai K et al. Enhanced elastin and fibrillin gene expression in chronically photodamaged skin. J Invest Dermatol 1994; 103: 182–6.
21. Fisher GJ, Wang Z, Datta SC et al. Pathophysiology of premature skin aging induced by ultraviolet light. New Engl J Med 1997; 337: 1419–28.
22. Frances C, Boisnic S, Hartmann DJ et al. Changes in the elastic tissue of the non-sun-exposed skin of cigarette smokers. Br J Dermatol 1991; 125: 43–7.
23. Kligman AM, Grove GL, Hirose R et al. Topical tretinoin for photoaged skin. J Am Acad Dermatol 1986; 15: 838–59.
24. Weinstein GD, Nigra TP, Pochi PE et al. Topical tretinoin for treatment of photodamaged skin. A multicentre study. Arch Dermatol 1991; 127: 659–65.
25. Sendagorta E, Lesiewicz J, Armstrong RB. Topical isotretinoin for photodamaged skin. J Am Acad Dermatol 1992; 27: 515–18.
26. Kang S, Krueger GG, Tanghetti EA et al. A multicenter randomized double blind trial of tazarotene 0.1% cream in the treatment of photodamage. J Am Acad Dermatol 2005; 52: 268–72.
27. Olsen EA, Katz HI, Levine N et al. Tretinoin emollient cream: a new therapy for photodamaged skin. J Am Acad Dermatol 1992; 26: 215–24.

Autoimmune disorders

The autoimmune group of disorders (sometimes known as autoaggressive diseases and which were previously also known as the connective tissue diseases) comprises lupus erythematosus, scleroderma, dermatomyositis and mixed connective tissue disease. Each of these 'polar' diseases includes several clinical types and may exhibit features of other of the polar disorders ('overlap' diseases). If this is not confusing enough it is also the case that other diseases such as the bullous disorders, vitiligo and alopecia areata also have an autoimmune pathogenesis. In any event in this chapter I will concentrate on the facial aspects of lupus erythematosus – scleroderma and dermatomyositis – and discuss their systemic aspects only briefly.

Lupus erythematosus

Lupus erythematosus (LE) is a not uncommon autoaggressive disorder in which various organs and tissues are the target of an immunological assault. The initiating events are uncertain but may involve viral infection, solar damage or both. Certainly damage to DNA with its subsequent release from the intracellular environment into the systemic circulation seems to play a role. The disorder includes a number of different types of disease which range from systemic LE (SLE), a multisystem and potentially fatal disease, to chronic discoid LE (CDLE), a persistent or recurrent inflammatory scarring disorder affecting sun-exposed skin.

Systemic lupus erythematosus and facial skin

The skin is affected in SLE in up to 70% patients at some point in their disease and the face is affected in the large majority of these.[1] Other areas of skin affected are the V of the neck and the dorsa of the hands and forearms, i.e. other light-exposed sites. Involvement of facial skin usually occurs early in the course of the disease alongside systemic symptoms before the development of arthropathy.

In some patients the condition develops after an episode of sun exposure or after some minor infective disorder such as an upper respiratory tract infection. 'Emotional turmoil' and other forms of stress are often blamed as the precipitating event but the relationship is notoriously difficult to prove.

Affected skin is at first red and slightly swollen, often involving the cheeks and the adjoining nasal skin giving the classical 'butterfly rash' appearance (Figure 8.1). Later the area may become irregularly atrophied and it then takes on the appearance of CDLE (see later). The differential diagnoses include rosacea, seborrheic dermatitis and dermatomyositis.

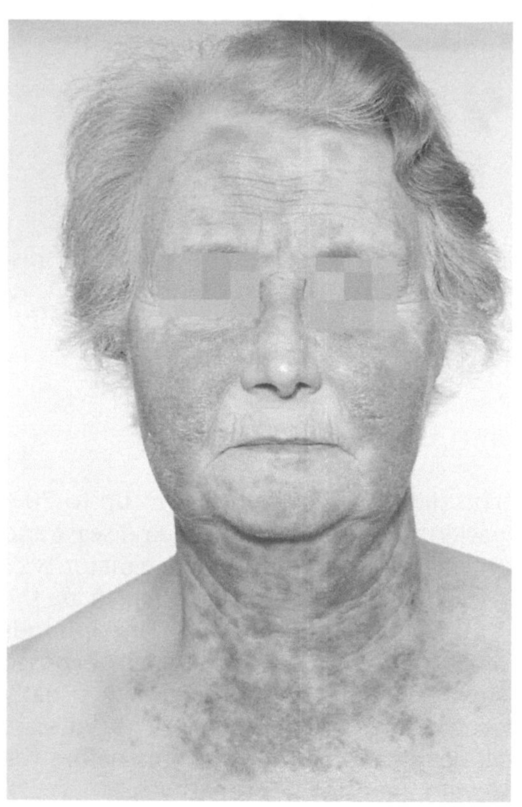

Figure 8.1

Systemic lupus erythematosus. Note the butterfly distribution of rash affecting either cheek and the bridge of the nose.

Pink hemispherical papules strongly support the diagnosis of the former common skin problem – although, confusingly, papules are rarely also seen in LE. The absence of systemic signs, symptoms and laboratory evidence also support a diagnosis of rosacea.

Scaling and flexural involvements suggest seborrheic dermatitis while a mauvish hue (heliotrope), involvement of the periocular skin and muscular aches, tenderness and weakness all suggest dermatomyositis.

Dermatopathology

The main features are a perivascular lymphocytic infiltrate and marked dermal edema. There is, in addition, in a substantial proportion of cases, basal cell liquefactive degenerative change. Staining with periodic acid – Schiff reagent reveals that the so-called 'basement membrane' is markedly thickened. This latter observation is related to the deposition of IgG and complement component C3 found at the dermoepidermal junction by direct immunofluorescence (IMF) tests. Positive IMF findings may also be found in normal-appearing skin of some 70% patients with SLE.[2]

Laboratory tests

Lymphopenia, neutropenia, thrombocytopenic anemia, raised ESR and hypergammaglobulinemia are amongst the many positive laboratory findings observed in patients with SLE. A positive antinuclear factor test is present in most patients and anti-double-stranded DNA antibodies, in high titer, are present in virtually all patients with SLE.[3]

Treatment

This will depend on the extent and severity of the disease, the organ systems affected and the functional problems that arise from these problems. Systemic corticosteroids, immunosuppressive agents and immunomodulatory biological agents are the major components in the treatment of SLE.

Chronic discoid lupus erythematosus (CDLE)

This disease is a chronic remittent destructive and scarring disorder of sun-exposed skin. Although CDLE does not regularly affect other organs or systems there is evidence of some systemic involvement in some patients with CDLE and the relationship between SLE and CDLE is far from clear. There is little doubt that a few patients with CDLE develop symptoms and signs of SLE. The rate of transformation of patients with CDLE into SLE is relatively low with reports varying from 1.3% per annum[4] to as high as 6–7% per annum.[5]

Many patients with CDLE have one or more positive laboratory tests that are more typical of SLE than a disorder supposedly confined to the skin, yet are asymptomatic.

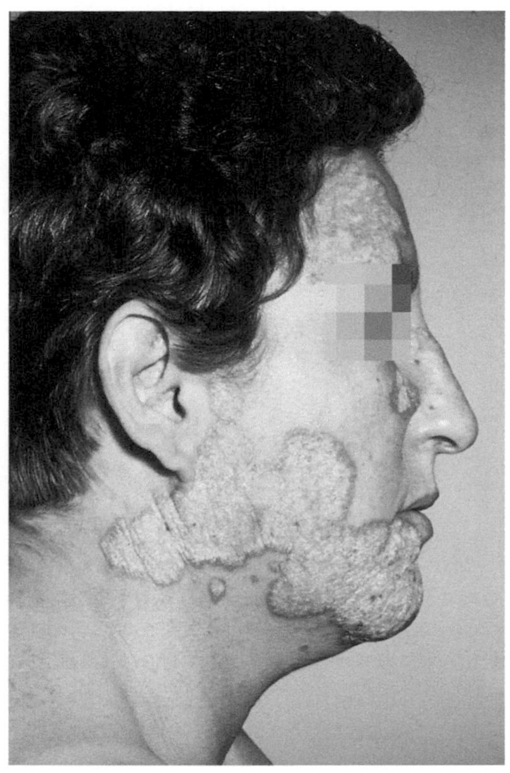

Figure 8.2

Chronic discoid lupus erythematosus (CDLE). There is a red scaling irregular plaque affecting the right cheek in this patient due to CDLE.

Clinical features

Irregularly thickened red plaques with well-defined margins develop on the face, neck, scalp and occasionally over the forearms (Figure 8.2). Certainly light exposure is an important localizing stimulus.[6] After a variable period, areas of atrophy and even scarring (Figure 8.2a) appear in the affected sites as do areas of dyspigmentation with both hyperpigmentation and hypopigmentation. Follicular orifices may become dilated and filled with horny plugs – the so-called 'tin tack sign'. Sometimes the affected sites may develop considerable hyperkeratosis and wartiness.

CDLE lesions affect patients over many years, the lesions becoming inflamed and quiescent alternately until eventually the disease seems to burn out.

One variant of CDLE is known as disseminated discoid lupus erythematosus (DDLE). The individual lesions are identical with CDLE but instead of there being 2–4 affected areas there may be 20–30.[7] In addition, the lesions seem to some extent 'synchronized' in that they tend to occur in batches.

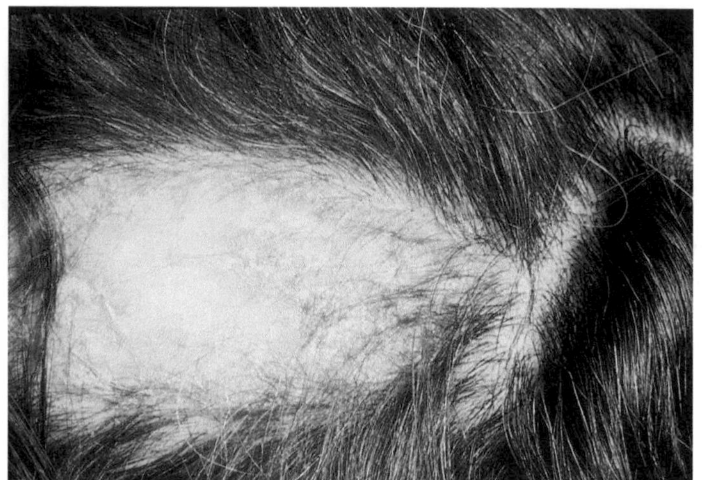

Figure 8.2a

Scarring alopecia due to CDLE. The affected area is red and scaly and shows complete loss of scalp hair.

These patients appear more 'unstable' than do patients with CDLE and transform to SLE very much more frequently than do patients with ordinary CDLE.

Skin pathology

In CDLE, basal layer liquefactive degenerative change is prominent and staining with periodic acid – Schiff reagent demonstrates a thickened mauve/purple bandin the subepidermal zone. This zone also stains for IgG and C3 by direct immunofluorescence. The epidermis is irregularly thickened and hyperkeratotic – though atrophy is seen later in the disease. There is a marked lymphocytic infiltrate in the dermis that is predominantly perivascular but also periadnexal (Figure 8.3).

Subacute lupus erythematosus

This condition was recognized as a subset of LE in 1979.[8] Some 80% of patients have anti-Ro SSA antibodies present and 60% have homogeneous antinuclear antibodies.

The skin lesions are more extensive than in CDLE and seem to involve the skin of the neck, the upper trunk and the upper arms in particular. The lesions may be red, papular and scaling or are annular and polycyclic. They may be vesicular or exudative at their margins. About half the patients have systemic involvement with fever, arthropathy and a pneumonitis.

Liquefactive degenerative change is more prominent histologically in subacute LE than in CDLE and colloid bodies are not uncommon.

Treatment of CDLE

All patients should be warned to avoid sun exposure and to use sunscreens. First-line treatment is with potent topical corticosteroids. Care must be taken to ensure that skin atrophy does not result. Intracutaneous injection with triamcinolone

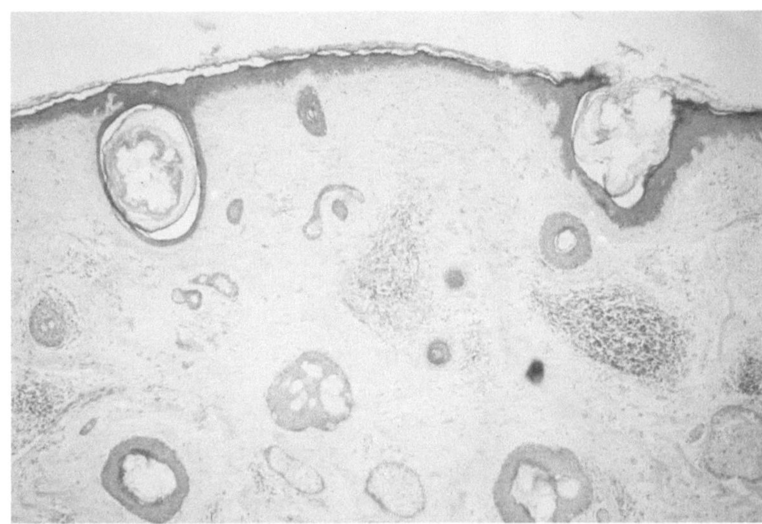

Figure 8.3

Photomicrograph of biopsy from patch of CDLE. Note the perivascular lymphocytic 'cuffing'.

acetonide or methylprednisolone may be used for thickened hyperkeratotic areas though great care has be taken to avoid too much or too superficial an injection in order to avoid unacceptable skin atrophy. If corticosteroids do not help, the antimalarial hydroxychloroquine by mouth (up to 400 mg daily) is effective for many patients. The drug has the uncommon but unpleasant adverse side effect of causing a retinal macular dystrophy and should not be continued for longer than a year. Checks by an ophthalmologist before starting and at 6-monthly intervals while on the drug are an important precaution. Mepacrine has also been employed, as has dapsone. The oral retinoids (e.g. acitretin) have been shown to be quite effective in suppressing CDLE[9] though not all patients consider the side effects and the necessary regular monitoring a worthwhile exchange for suppression of the disorder. Oral gold preparations ('auranofin') are helpful for some patients with recalcitrant disease.[10]

Thalidomide has also been successfully used for some patients.[11]

Scleroderma

Included in this category are morphea (localized scleroderma), systemic sclerosis and generalized morphea. They are probably all autoimmune disorders which share pathogenetic pathways.

Systemic sclerosis (SS)

This is a serious generalized disorder affecting the kidneys, the lungs, the gastro-intestinal tract, the vasculature and the skin (only the facial changes will be described here).

The face in SS shows quite characteristic features (Figure 8.4). When well developed, the features seem 'pinched' or bird-like with thinning of the nose and hollowing of the cheeks as well as a

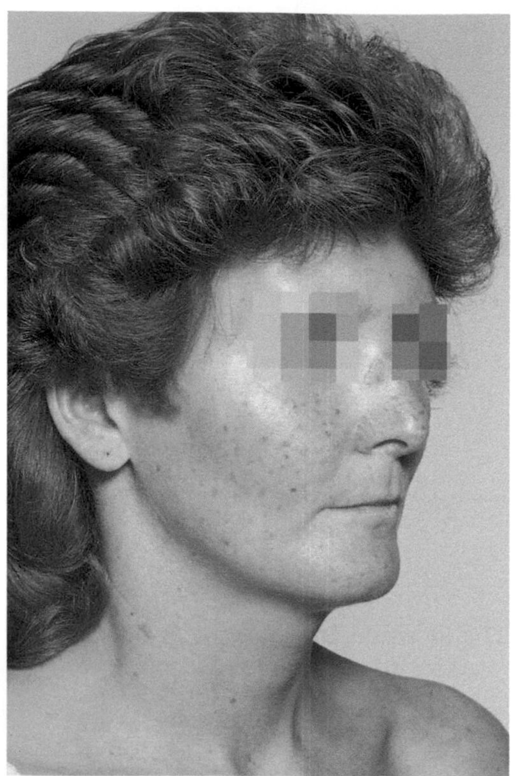

Figure 8.4

The face in systemic sclerosis. The mouth is reduced in size (microstomia), the nose is thin and prominent, the cheeks are sunken and the skin smooth and atrophic.

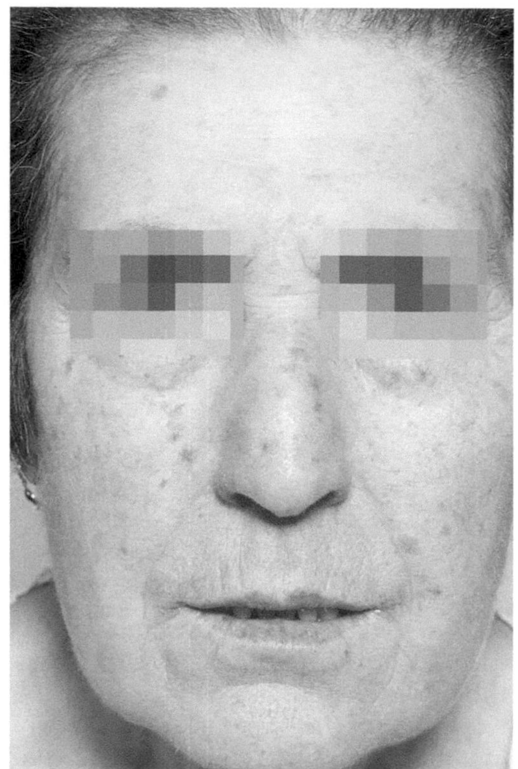

Figure 8.5

There are telangiectatic macules on the cheeks of this patient with systemic sclerosis.

background pallor. The lips tend to be thin, framing a mouth that is reduced in size (microstomia). 'Star-like' telangiectatic macules occur over the cheeks and forehead (Figure 8.5). These alterations often occur alongside 'acrosclerosis' with changes in the hands and forearms.[12]

Morphea

Morphea is also known as localized scleroderma. The face is not often involved in ordinary morphea but is affected by a special and somewhat curious atrophic disorder known by the colorful name of 'en coup de sabre' (Figure 8.6). In this condition there is an area of skin and muscle atrophy starting at the chin and spreading upward over the face in a pattern fancifully likened to the effects of a sabre blow. The condition affects adolescents and young adults in particular and after a period of worsening becomes static and persistent.

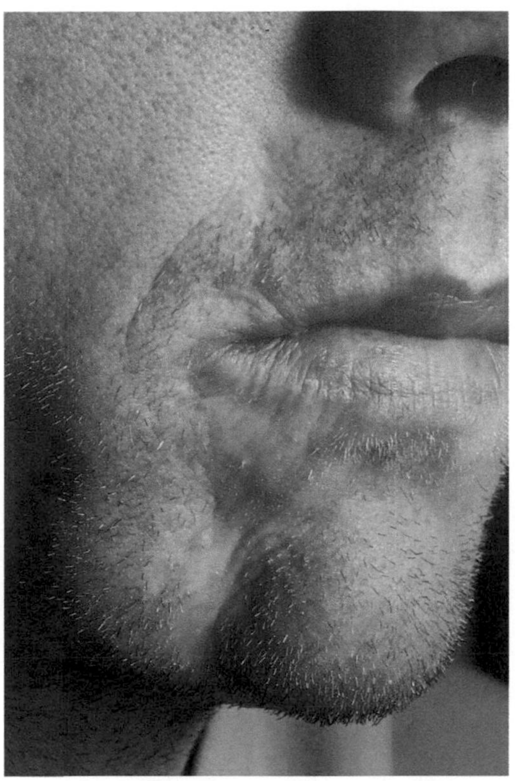

Figure 8.6

Facial deformity due to the condition of facial morphea known as 'en coup de sabre'.

Generalized morphea

In this very uncommon disorder, the skin is affected by stiffening, slight swelling and a mauve-pink discoloration or lividity. The condition usually starts on the face or upper chest and gradually spreads all over the trunk and limbs. Unfortunately the chest wall is often so badly affected that respiratory movements become impossible so that respiratory assistance is required.

Pathology of scleroderma

The most dramatic of the histological alterations is the change in the dermal collagen which is most evident in a recently appearing patch of morphea. The collagenous tissue is paler staining than usual and appears 'glassy' or 'homogenized'. Furthermore, there seems to be more dermal collagen than in normal skin and in fact the skin is thicker than usual.[13] This odd-looking dermal connective tissue extends downwards into the subcutaneous fat and appears to have been recently formed. In addition there is a variably intense perivascular lymphocytic infiltrate especially in the lower parts of the dermis. The question as to what fires off the fibroblasts to produce new collagen inappropriately is unsolved but seems to be lymphocyte driven.[14]

Treatment of scleroderma

Currently there is no predictably effective method of halting the progress of the disease in any of its manifestations. Some success has been claimed for immunosuppressive agents and/or steroids but the evidence that this is helpful is very slim.[15] Claims of a beneficial effect of oral D-penicillamine in morphea should be accepted with caution – any improvement noted is of a minor degree.

Dermatomyositis

This is an uncommon autoaggressive disorder which affects both skin and muscle although in a few cases only muscle appears to be involved (polymyositis) and in an even smaller number of patients it is only the skin that is affected. The myositis predominantly involves the proximal limb girdle muscles and is first noted as weakness and tenderness over the affected muscles. Difficulties in sitting up from the recumbent position and the acts of combing and brushing the hair are classically amongst the first problems complained of by patients. Later in the disease the muscle weakness may become profound and generalized and may affect the respiratory and pharyngeal muscles – then becoming life-threatening.

The skin involvement is variable – the skin of the face being affected in the majority of patients. Other sites affected include the backs of the hands and the dorsa of the fingers, the paronychial skin of the fingers, the elbows and the knees and, in the worst cases, scattered areas over the trunk. Affected sites are dull red in color and slightly swollen. The upper part of the face is characteristically affected (Figure 8.7) by a mauvish erythema – so-called heliotrope in color. The periocular tissues are swollen as well as discolored giving a distinctive appearance. On the hands the erythematous areas over the dorsa of the fingers are known as 'Gottron's papules'. The paronychial skin is erythematous and the eponychium becomes irregularly thickened (or ragged). Viewed with a strong magnifying glass, irregularly enlarged capillaries can be seen in the nail bed.

The differential diagnosis of the facial rash includes rosacea and lupus erythematosus. The diagnosis can be confirmed by laboratory investigations[16,17] including the blood level of muscle enzymes, the urinary excretion of creatine and the histological appearances of muscle biopsy – showing up focal degenerative changes and lymphocytic infiltration. Electromyography may also reveal characteristic changes.

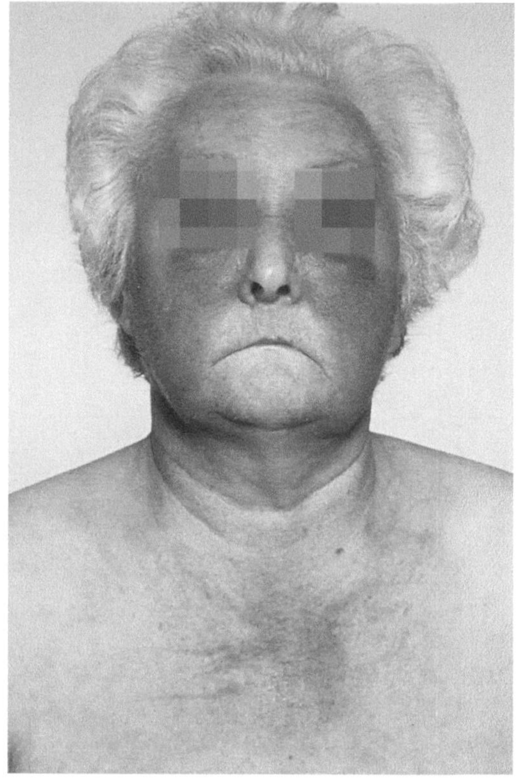

Figure 8.7

This lady has dermatomyositis. The facial rash is most prominent around the eyes and often has a mauve (or heliotrope) discoloration.

The relationship of the onset of dermatomyositis to underlying neoplastic disease has been debated over many years.[18,19] It appears that in women over the age of 40 there is a 50% chance of there being an ovarian or genital tract neoplasm in patients with dermatomyositis. A particular relationship has also been claimed for gastrointestinal tumors.

The treatment of dermatomyositis is with systemic steroids and immunosuppressive agents.

References

1. Patel P, Werth V. Cutaneous lupus erythematosus: a review. Dermatol Clin 2002; 20: 373–85.
2. Tuffanelli D. Cutaneous immunopathology: recent observations. J Invest Dermatol 1975; 65: 143–53.
3. Alarcon-Segovia D. The pathogenesis of immune dysregulation in systemic lupus erythematosus. A troika. J Rheumatol 1984; 11: 588–90.
4. Rowell NR. Laboratory abnormalities in the diagnosis and management of lupus erythematosus. Br J Dermatol 1971; 84: 210–16.
5. Millard LG, Rowell NR, Rajah SM. Histocompatability antigens in discoid and systemic lupus erythematosus. Br J Dermatol 1977; 96: 139–44.
6. Epstein JH, Tuffanelli DL, Dubois DL. Light sensitivity and lupus erythematosus. Arch Dermatol 1965; 91: 482.
7. Goodfield MJD, James SK, Veale DJ. In: Burns DA, Breathnach S, Cox N et al, eds. Textbook of Dermatology, 7th edn. Oxford: Blackwell, 2004: The connective tissue diseases 56.11.
8. Sontheimer RD, Thomas JR, Gilliam JN. Subacute cutaneous lupus erythematosus. Arch Dermatol 1979; 115: 1409–15.
9. Ruzicka T, Sommarburg C, Bieber T. Efficiency of acitretin in the treatment of cutaneous lupus erythematosus. Arch Dermatol 1988; 124: 897–902.
10. Dalziel K, Going S, Cartwright PH et al. Treatment of chronic lupus erythematosus with an oral gold compound (Auranofin). Br J Dermatol 1986; 115: 211–16.
11. Knop J, Bonomann G, Happle R et al. Thalidomide in the treatment of 60 cases of chronic discoid lupus erythematosus. Br J Dermatol 1983; 108: 461–6.
12. Jacobsen F, Halberg P, Ullman S et al. Clinical features and serum antinuclear antibodies in 230 Danish patients with systemic sclerosis. Br J Rheumatol 1998; 37: 39–45.
13. Akesson A, Hasselsrand R, Scheja A et al. Longitudinal development of skin involvement and reliability of high frequency ultrasound in systemic sclerosis. Ann Rheum Dis 2004; 63: 791–8.
14. Sato S. [B_4 cell abnormalities and autoantibody production in systemic sclerosis]. Nikon Rinsho Meneki Gakkai Kaishi 2006; 29: 73–84.
15. Choy E, Hoogendijk J, Lecky B et al. Immunosuppressant and immunomodulatory treatment for dermatomyositis and polymyositis. Cochrane Database Syst Rev 2005; (3): CD003643.
16. Brown VE, Pilkington CA, Feldman BM, Davidson JE. An international consensus survey of the diagnostic criteria for juvenile dermatomyositis (JDM). Rheumatology (Oxford). 2006; 45: 990–3.
17. Genth E. Inflammatory muscle diseases. Dermatomyositis polymyositis and inclusion body myositis. Internist (Berl.) 2005; 46: 1218–32.
18. Cherin P, Piette JC, Herson S. Dermatomyositis and ovarian cancer: a report of 7 cases and literature review. J Rheumatol 1993; 11: 1897–9.
19. Gainon J, Bart PA, Waeber G. Can we predict the risk of malignancy associated with dermatomyositis? Schwertz Rundsch Med Praxis 2003; 92: 1734–9.

Tumors of facial skin

This chapter will deal with neoplastic lesions that occur exclusively, predominantly or very frequently on facial skin. Skin cancer is increasingly common because of increased leisure time, increased access to holidays in the sun and an overwhelming desire (difficult to understand) to look sun-tanned. The face is a particular target for solar damage and neoplasms that develop after prolonged exposure to ultraviolet radiation are especially common on the face. In addition the large number of well-developed hair follicles and sebaceous glands also influence the type of lesion seen in this region. It has been computed, for example, that the incidence of treated non-melanoma skin cancer in Australia in 2002 was more than 5 times the incidence of all other cancers combined.[1]

Epithelial tumors

Seborrheic keratoses (seborrheic warts, basal cell papillomata)

Like barnacles on a rusting ship these common and benign tumors accumulate on the skin with increasing age. They occur virtually anywhere on the skin but are frequently found on the upper trunk, the face and the backs of the hands. On the face they are often seen on the temples, forehead and preauricular regions. On facial skin they tend to be less warty and thickened than on the trunk (Figures 9.1a and 9.1b). Seborrheic keratoses are usually a shade of brown but vary from 'skin-colored' through fawn to black. They need to be distinguished from other flat pigmented lesions including senile lentigo, lentigo maligna and

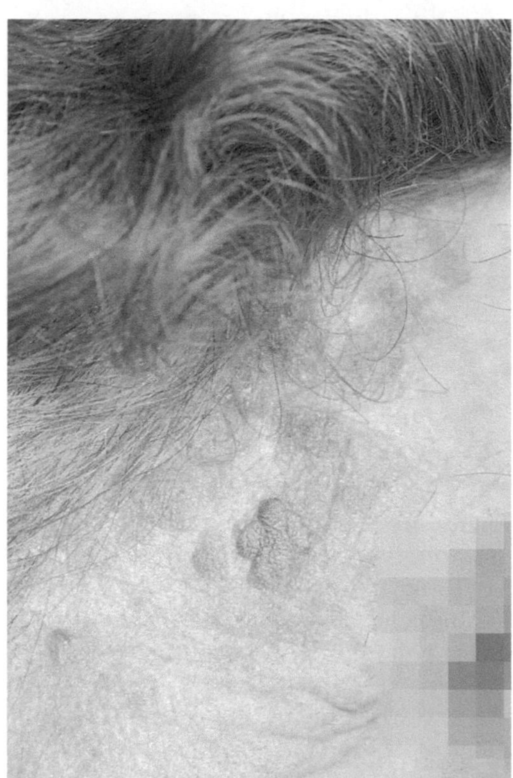

Figure 9.1a

Light brown and fawn seborrheic warts affecting the temple.

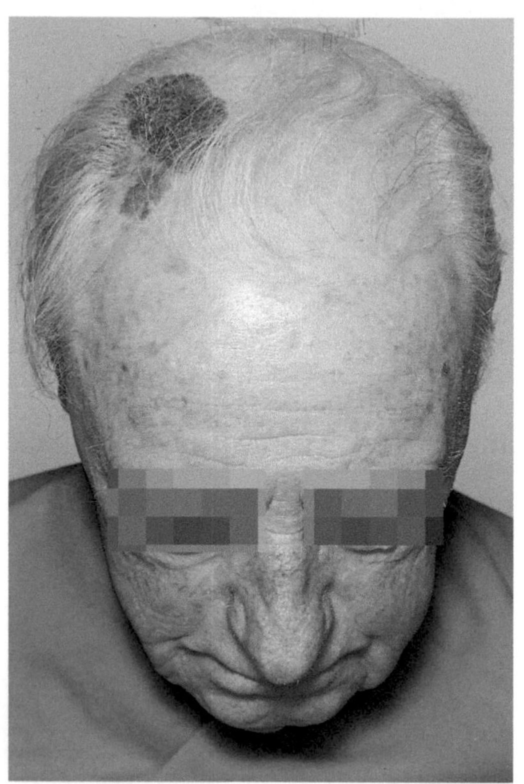

Figure 9.1b

Seborrheic wart on scalp.

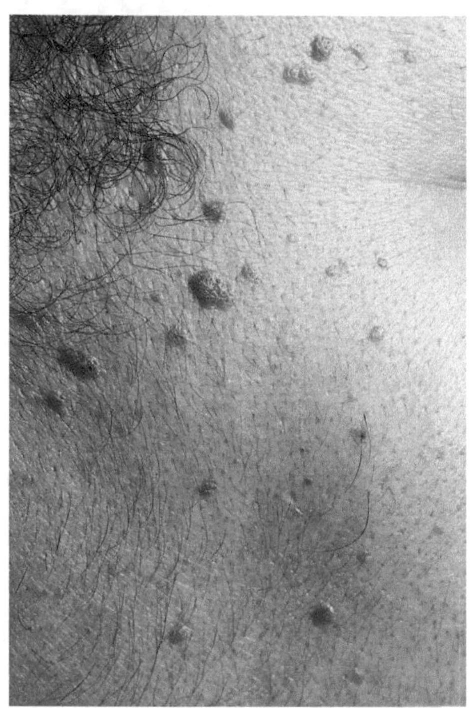

Figure 9.1c

Black papular lesions known as dermatosis papulosa nigra. These are the equivalent of facial seborrheic warts in dark-skinned subjects.

pigmented basal cell carcinoma. Ordinary lentigines are completely flat and uniform in color. Patients with lentigo maligna usually say that the lesion has been enlarging and becoming irregularly darker. In dark-skinned patients seborrheic warts tend to be black and papular (Figure 9.1c) and are then known as dermatosis papulosa nigra.

Pathology

Seborrheic warts consist of immature 'basaloid keratinocytes'. In places there are attempts at keratinization with foci of horn forming within swirls of keratinocytes – known as 'squamous eddies'. The surface is warty and irregular and may be 'church steeple'-like (Figures 9.2a and 9.2b). There are deep crypts between the horny spires. The whole lesion often appears 'stuck on' to the skin surface.

Treatment

Treatment is only indicated if the lesions cause symptoms, cause cosmetic

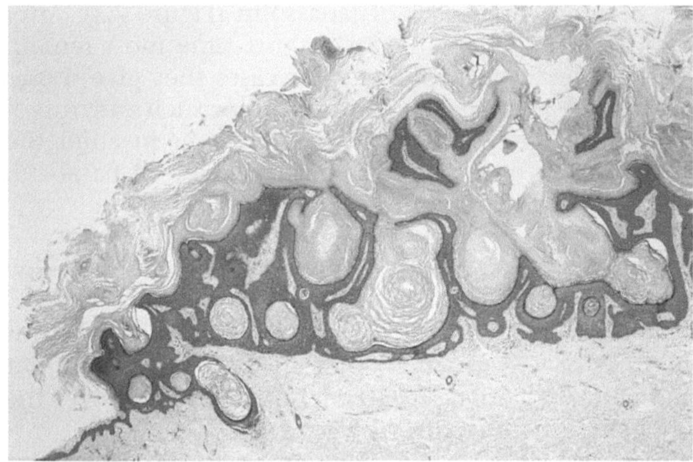

Figure 9.2a

Photomicrograph of seborrheic wart. Note the 'stuck on' appearance (hematoxylin and eosin × 25).

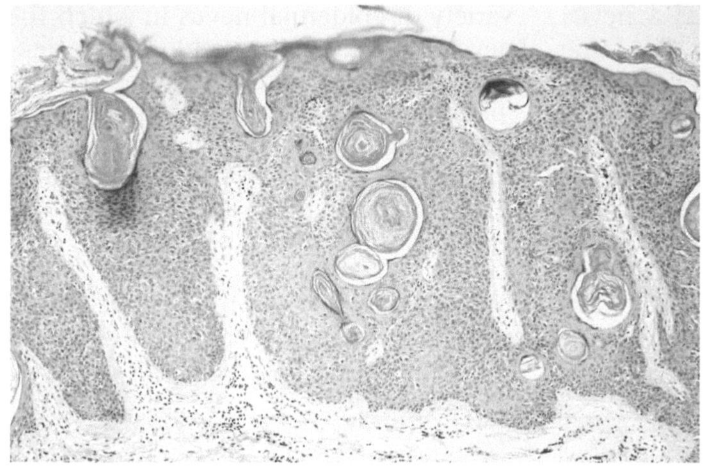

Figure 9.2b

Histology of seborrheic wart showing many horn cysts (hematoxylin and eosin × 45).

embarrassment, get in the way or there is doubt as to diagnosis. The most effective treatment is to remove them by curettage (under a local anesthetic) with light cautery subsequently. Cryotherapy with liquid nitrogen is quicker and easier for the operator but more painful and less effective. Where there are large numbers of lesions treatment may have to be spread over several sessions. Groups of small lesions can be treated with 2% salicylic acid in white soft paraffin twice daily as this will keep them small and unobtrusive.

Inverted follicular keratosis

This is an uncommon crateriform lesion occurring predominantly on the face and around the nose in partricular[2]. They are probably a type of seborrheic wart[3] and consist of benign epilthelial masses with the histological characteristics of an irritated seborrheic wart and foci of horn formation. There is a central horny plug although the major part of the abnormal epithelium is below the general level of the epidermis. They are rarely recognized prior to their removal.

Epidermal nevus; nevus sebaceus of Jadassohn; comedone nevus

These congenital malformations are hamartomata and consist of benign inappropriate proliferations of admixtures of warty epidermal hyperplasia and abnormally situated enlarged sebaceous glands, eccrine and apocrine sweat ducts and glands. If the sebaceous element predominates the lesion is known as a nevus sebaceus but it is essentially the same type of lesion.[4]

Warty epidermal nevus can occur anywhere on the skin but it is quite often found on the face and scalp. Lesions with more sebaceous glands on them tend to occur on the scalp where they are noted at birth or shortly thereafter. They have an orange color and are known as nevus sebaceus of Jadassohn (Figure 9.3). After enlarging for a short time most remain static but in some cases they give rise to a benign adnexal tumor such as syringocystadenoma papilliferum. In adult life they sometimes give rise to a basal cell carcinoma.

It should be noted that some warty nevi are linear and curiously psoriasiform.[5,6] These are known as inflammatory linear verrucous epidermal nevus (ILVEN) but appear to be mainly distributed over the lower trunk and legs.

Comedone nevus may be considered a variety of epidermal nevus in which the developmental defect resides in the genesis of the follicular structures so that 'blind follicular canals' are formed giving rise to comedones. Of interest with regard to the pathogenesis of acne is the fact that inflammatory acne-type lesions sometimes form in these lesions.

Becker's nevus[7] in which there is hyperplasia of many of the epidermal elements

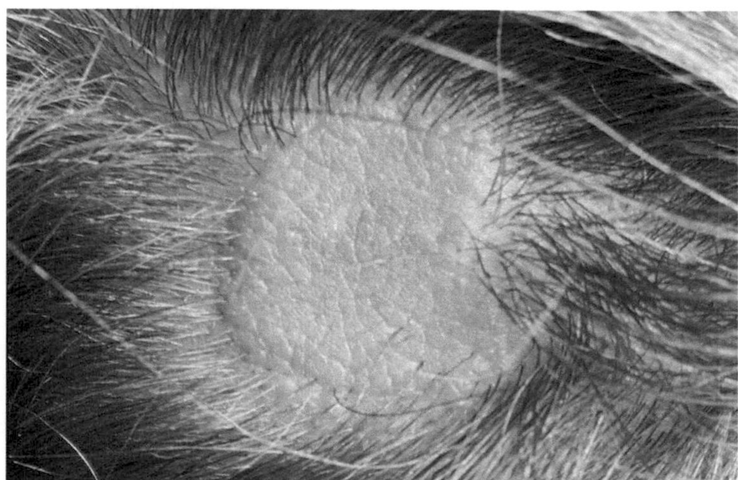

Figure 9.3

Orange warty plaque on scalp of 12-year-old boy. Typical of nevus sebaceus of Jadassohn.

as well as hyperpigmentation occurring over a limb girdle is also a variety of epidermal nevus. In this disorder slightly thickened and pigmented hairy skin covers one shoulder and upper arm or more uncommonly the buttock and thigh.

Epidermal nevus is also a concomitant of a number of congenital syndromes[8] with diverse clinical components.

Treatment

Where indicated, and feasible, removal by surgery or laser ablation is indicated.

Syringomata

These are benign sweat gland tumors which are virtually always multiple. They are more common in women and occur predominantly on the face – on the eyelids, upper cheeks and neck (Figure 9.4). Uncommonly they have a much wider distribution, developing over the trunk and limbs quite rapidly. In one study[9] it was found that of the 35 cases of syringomata studied all had lesions on the face while 70% had lesions on the limbs and trunk. Syringomata are small (2–4 mm diameter), skin-colored, white or pink papules which may appear lichenoid and are mistaken for lichen planus. They are generally asymptomatic.

Pathology

Characteristically, there are multiple small irregular tubules and cysts (often comma-shaped) in the upper and mid dermis. These are lined by a double row of cuboidal basophilic cells. Sometimes the 'microcysts' contain amorphous material and at others the contents consist of concentric lamellae of horn.

The consensus is that these lesions are apocrine in origin but one study in which the author was involved suggested that they might be derived from primitive cells which can also show differentiation towards hair follicle structures.

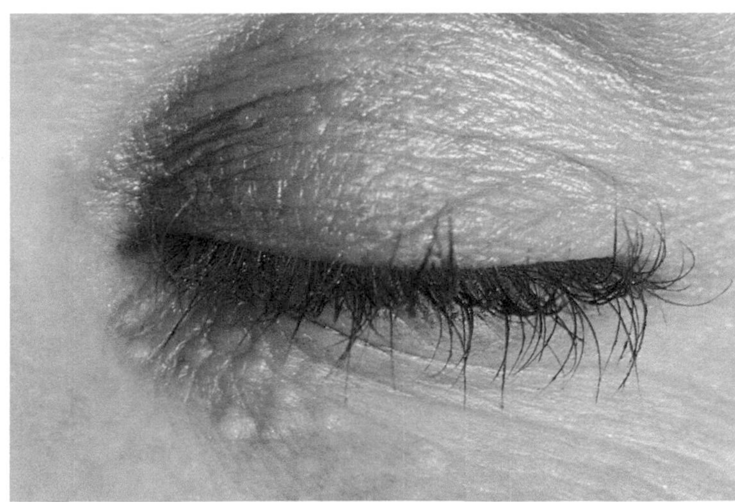

Figure 9.4

Lesions of syringoma.

Treatment

Individual lesions can be removed by surgery, cautery or laser ablation.

Trichoepithelioma (epithelioma adenoides cysticum)

These uncommon benign tumors of hair follicles may be solitary or multiple. They are small, skin-coloured or pearly nodules. If single they may occur anywhere on the face and may resemble nodulocystic basal cell carcinoma. When multiple they tend to develop symmetrically over the cheeks and may be mistaken for syringomata although unlike syringomata they do not cluster around the eyes. The condition appears heritable as an autosomal dominant characteristic.

Pathology

There are clumps and nodules of basaloid cells and cysts containing horny debris. Other than the cysts they look quite like basal cell carcinoma.

Pilomatricoma (calcifying epithelioma of Malherbe)

This not uncommon lesion arises from the hair follicle matrix. They may occur at any age but are quite common in the young. In one study 45% of 179 lesions occurred in patients aged 18 or less.[10] Clinically, lesions are usually single, firm or hard, skin-colored or slightly bluish nodules occuring on the face, neck and shoulders. A syndrome has been described in which these lesions are inherited, together with the symptom complex known as myotonic dystrophy.[11]

Pathology

Interestingly the basaloid epithelium in these tumors undergoes a special kind of necrosis, eventual calcification and even ossification. The cells in the calcified tissue can still be identified in outline and are known as 'ghost cells' (Figure 9.5).

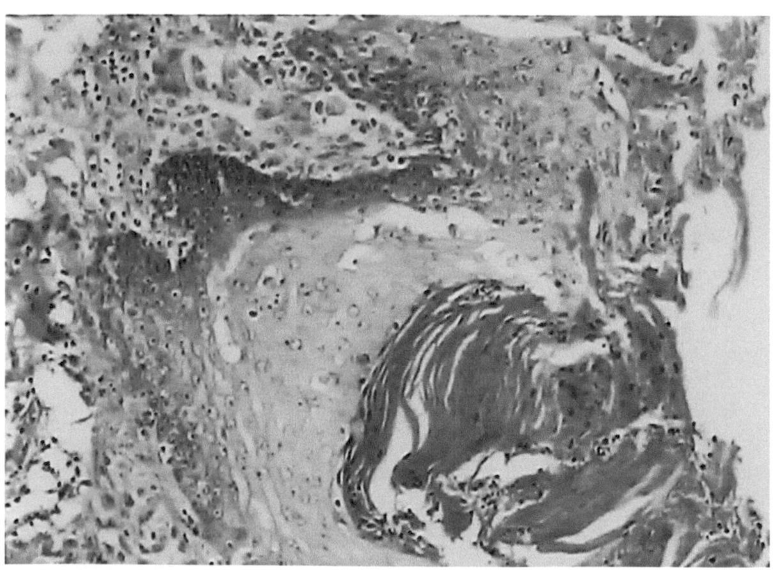

Figure 9.5

Photomicrograph from sample of pilomatricoma. There are basaloid cells around an area of transformation containing 'ghost cells' (hematoxylin and eosin × 150).

Sebaceous gland neoplasms

True neoplasms of the sebaceous glands are very rare. A sebaceous adenoma does exist but is very uncommon compared to senile sebaceous gland hypertrophy.

Senile sebaceous gland hypertrophy

The cause of SSGH is quite mysterious, but results in the appearance of a number of small orange-yellow intracutaneous nodules (Figure 9.6), around the nose, cheeks and chin particularly. They are often mistaken for basal cell carcinoma. They are odd as they represent one of the few phenomena of hypertrophy in aging – mostly things get smaller!

Histologically considerably enlarged but otherwise normal sebaceous gland lobules are evident quite high up in the dermis. The section may appear to contain only sebaceous glands.

Trichofolliculoma and folliculoma

These are uncommon hamartomatous lesions of hair follicle epithelium which occur predominantly on the face as single intracutaneous nodules. The abnormal epithelium may mimic or caricature ordinary follicular structures.

Cylindroma ('turban tumors')

These are uncommon benign tumors of sweat gland epithelium. They occur as multiple nodules on the scalp and are frequently inherited as an autosomal dominant characteristic (Figure 9.7).

Pathology

The tumor consists of oval and rounded dermal aggregates of basaloid cells amongst which are a few larger and more eosinophilic cells (Figure 9.8). The surrounding connective tissue often has a pink hyaline quality which may also be seen to a lesser extent in certain other sweat gland tumors.

Syringocystadenoma papilliferum

This is a rare sweat gland tumor of apocrine origin. It occurs on the scalp or

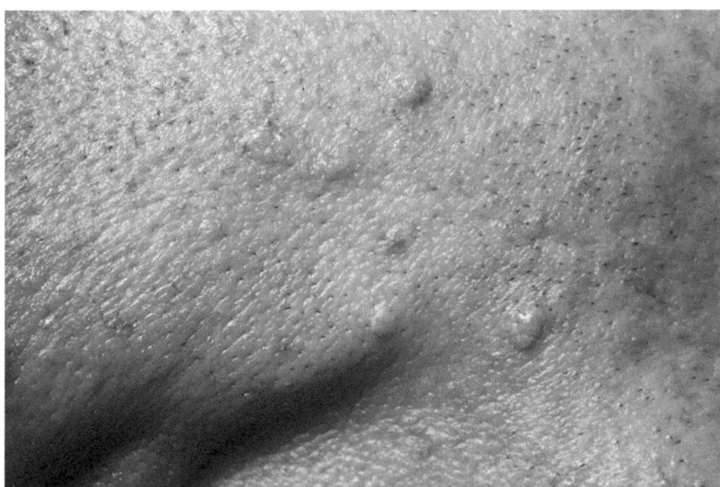

Figure 9.6

Senile sebaceous gland hypertrophy. These orange/skin-colored papules on the jaw are typical of this disorder.

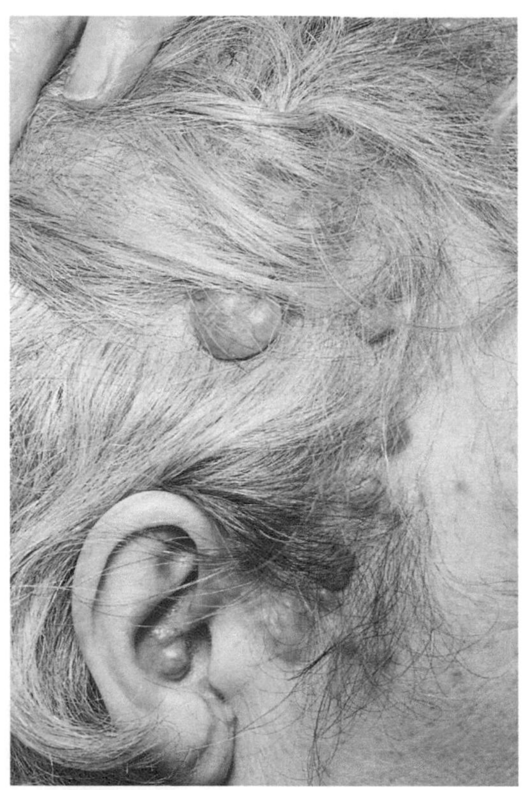

Figure 9.7

Multiple nodules in the scalp due to cylindroma.

in women in the perigenital area. It is usually a single skin-colored nodule with a 'pore' at the apex or may appear frond-like initially. They sometimes arise within a nevus sebaceus.

Pathology

They consist of two cell types in a characteristic villous or frond-like pattern. There are also many plasma cells present.

Hidrocystoma

This is an uncommon anomaly of apocrine structures. The lesion occurs exclusively on the face as a solitary bluish cystic structure which varies in size with the temperature. It is due to cystic dilatation of apocrine ducts as a result of a developmental anomaly or an obstruction. It is said to occur more frequently in washerwomen.

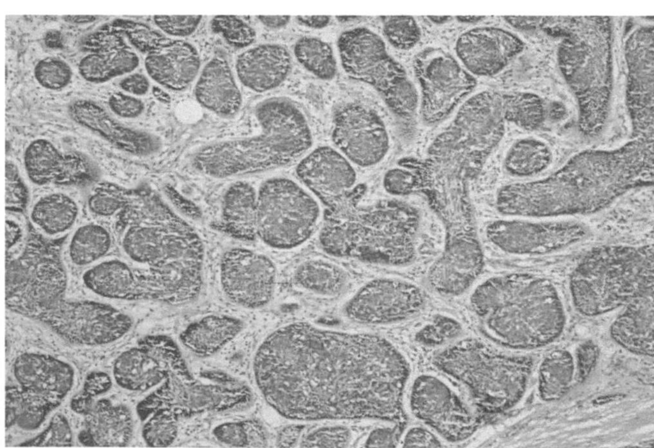

Figure 9.8

Histology of cylindroma. There are multiple nodules of basaloid cells which appear almost faceted together (hematoxylin and eosin $\times$ 30).

Malignant epithelial tumors

Basal cell carcinoma (basal cell epithelioma, rodent ulcer, BCC)

BCC is the most common malignant tumor in man. It affects Caucasians predominantly and is especially common in those who have been constantly exposed to the sun. It is especially common in fair-complexioned inhabitants of Australia, South Africa and the Southern United States.[12]

The lay term 'rodent ulcer' must have originated in the fancied likeness of the neglected large ulcerated nodules of BCC to rat bites. Luckily such lesions are rarely seen today!

Multiple BCC are also seen in the condition known as the basal cell nevus syndrome (Gorlin's syndrome) in which palmar pits, CNS tumors, mandibular cysts and other bony anomalies – such as bifid ribs may occur. The BCC in this odd genodermatosis are often pigmented. It is inherited as an autosomal dominant characteristic. BCC also arise in areas of previous radiotherapy.

Clinical appearance

Although more common in the elderly, BCC may also be seen in young adults – and are then often found to have arisen in epidermal nevi.

Most commonly they arise on the face, though over 30% occur in covered areas. Several types are recognized: nodulocystic, ulcerative, morpheic and pigmented. The nodulocystic type consists of afirm pink-grayish or pearly papule or nodule (Figure 9.9). This sort is notoriously slow-growing and because of this and the ease with which it is removed has the best prognosis. If they ulcerate they form superficial ulcers (ulcerative type) with rolled pearly margins (Figure 9.10). If these lesions affect the perinasal or periauricular area they may be difficult to eradicate because of their propensity to invade cartilage and may then cause very unpleasant destruction of areas of the face.

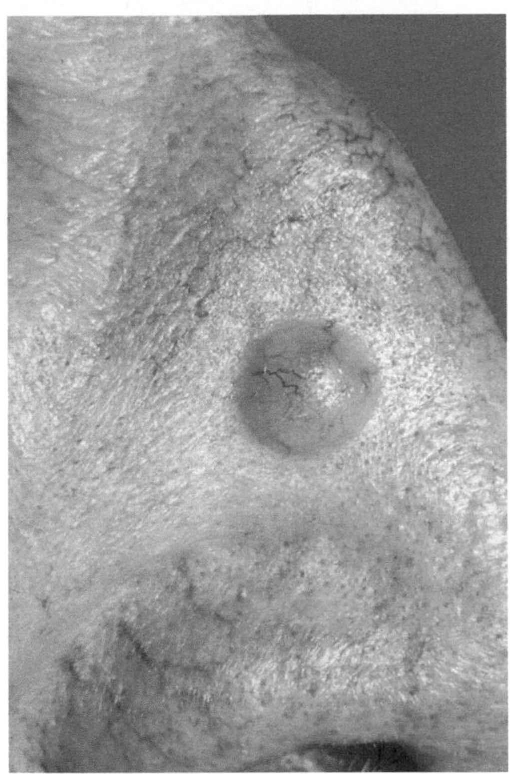

Figure 9.9

Nodulocystic basal cell carcinoma. This common type of BCC often has a 'pearly' appearance and not infrequently telangiectatic blood vessels course over the surface.

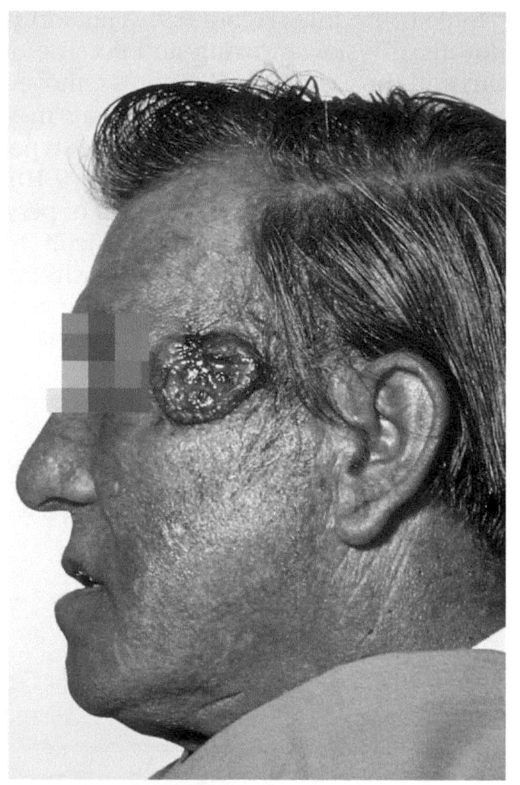

Figure 9.10

Large ulcerated nodule of BCC.

Pigmented BCC is a brown black variant of the nodulocystic type. They are often misdiagnosed as a melanocytic lesion of one sort or another (Figure 9.11).

Superficial BCC are quite often multiple and are more common on the trunk than on the face. They form pink slightly raised scaly irregular macules or plaques. Often the margin has a very thin but definitely rolled pearly edge.

The morpheic type of BCC causes indurated firm often depressed plaques or patches. There may be little in the way of surface change and they are infamous for the difficulties that they cause in diagnosis. Their extent may be difficult to define so that there is a danger that they are inadequately removed.

Pathology

All types consist of irregular clumps, columns and variously shaped aggregates of small basophilic cells (Figure 9.12).

There is varying stromal reaction with fibrosis which is particularly evident in

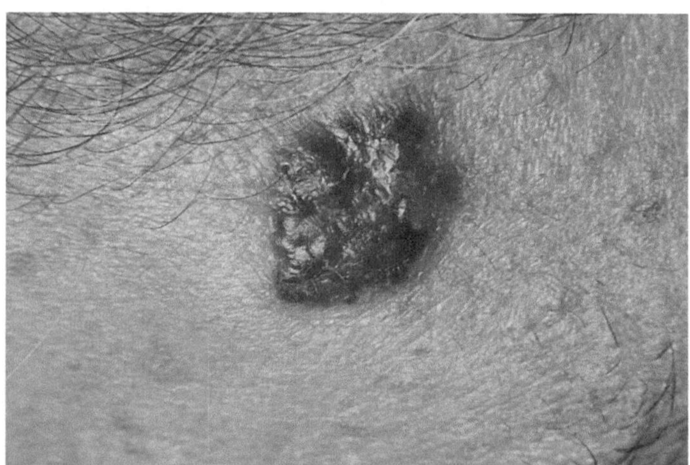

Figure 9.11

Pigmented BCC. These are often mistaken for melanocytic lesions.

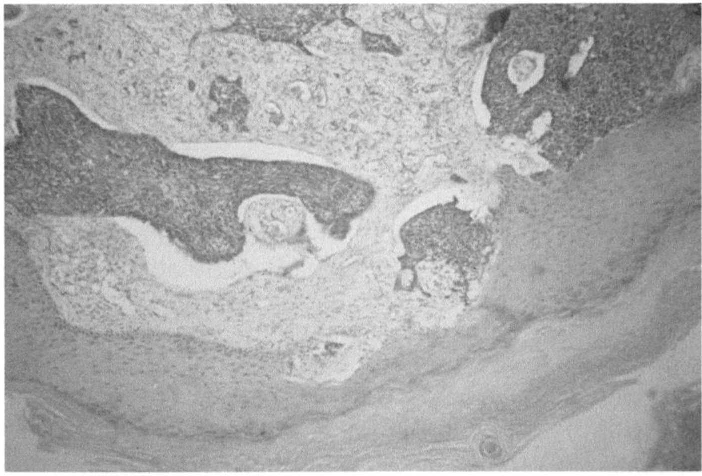

Figure 9.12

Histology of BCC. Clumps and nodules of basaloid cells in the dermis. They often have an artefictual 'space' around their periphery (hematoxylin and eosin × 30).

morpheic BCC. The cells at the margin of the clumps are often orientated perpendicularly to the tumor lobules giving an appearance of 'palisading'. There is often a degree of mucoid degeneration in the tumor either within the tumor lobules or at the margins of the lobules. This results in separation of the basaloid cells from the fibrous stroma in routinely prepared histological sections. The tumor lobules may have a very 'organized' look to them and on occasions appear to emulate pilar structures. This type of arrangement is associated with the least malignant potential.

Pathogenesis

There has been much work on the molecular mechanisms involved in the pathogenesis of BCC in recent years.[11] Mutations in p53 and the 'patched' gene – Hedgehog signaling system – as well as suppression of the cell hypersensitivity response are involved but the exact relationships have not as yet been elucidated.

Treatment

Surgical exicision is the most suitable treatment for most small lesions – save those where an unpleasant cosmetic result is likely to be obtained. Generally a margin of 3 mm around the lesion should be allowed. Small nodulocystic or superficial lesions are easily treated by curettage and cautery. The cosmetic result is surprisingly good. Care should be taken to remove all the tumorous tissue from the base and edges by repeating the stroke of the curette on two or three occasions before applying the cautery. The recurrence rate is higher than with excision but with care should not be more than 2–3%.

Large BCC lesions around the nose, eyes and ears require great care in surgical removal and should only be tackled by those with specialized knowledge and experience. Microsurgical techniques with microscopic monitoring of the tissue removed give the best results with the lowest recurrence rates.[13] Excellent results can also be obtained by using topical chemotherapeutic agents such as 5% 5-fluorouracil ointment (applied twice daily over a 14-day period) or 5% imiquimod used daily for 3 days per week. These chemotherapeutic methods are particularly suitable for large lesions in elderly patients who would not tolerate surgery very well. However, chemotherapy may cause considerable inflammation at the site of treatment.

In recent years another therapy has been developed dependent on the cytotoxic effect of photoactivated porphyrins in malignant cells. The affected site is treated with 5-aminolevulinic acid (or a derivative) and then irradiated with a beam of non-coherent light. This is known as photodynamic therapy and has been successfully used for all types of NMSC – including BCC.[14]

Radiotherapy is also a useful alternative for patients in whom surgery would be difficult or hazardous.

Prognosis

The vast majority of lesions are easily removed and most methods of treatment are associated with low recurrence rates of 1–3%. There are reports of metastasizing BCC but these are few and far between as the condition is so uncommon. Unfortunately there are no ways of distinguishing the rare lesions that do metastasize either clinically or histologically.[15]

Solar keratoses (senile keratoses, actinic keratoses, SK)

These are usually classified as premalignant but only a very small proportion actually transform into squamous cell carcinoma. They are extremely common – especially in sunny climates. Robin Marks, working in rural Queensland, Australia found that more than 50% of those over the age of 40 had SKs.[16] Our own studies in cool and comparatively sunless South Wales revealed surprisingly that some 23% of the population over 60 years of age had SKs.[17] A Merseyside population was also found to have a large number of SKs.[18] A surprisingly high proportion remit spontaneously. In the study by Robin Marks, 30% of the original lesions could no longer be identified after 1 year. In this study as well as our own it seems that less than one in 1000 transform into SCC.[19]

Clinical features

They are found on all light-exposed sites – particularly the face, the V of the neck, the ears, the backs of the hands and the bald area of the scalp. They also occur on the lower legs in women (presumably due to the custom of wearing a skirt). They are mostly slightly raised, pink or gray scaling patches 2–6 mm in diameter (Figure 9.13). Occasionally they are pinker and larger and then look CDLE-like (see page 115) – so-called lupoid keratoses. Another uncommon presentation is as a cutaneous horn (Figure 9.14).

Pathology

The hallmark of the SK is that the keratinocytes 'look different' in that they are irregular in size, shape and staining reaction. They also possess nuclei that are irregular in size and shape and which show abnormal mitoses. These abnormal cells are often irregularly orientated compared to the normal epidermis and the affected epidermis is surmounted by parakeratosis

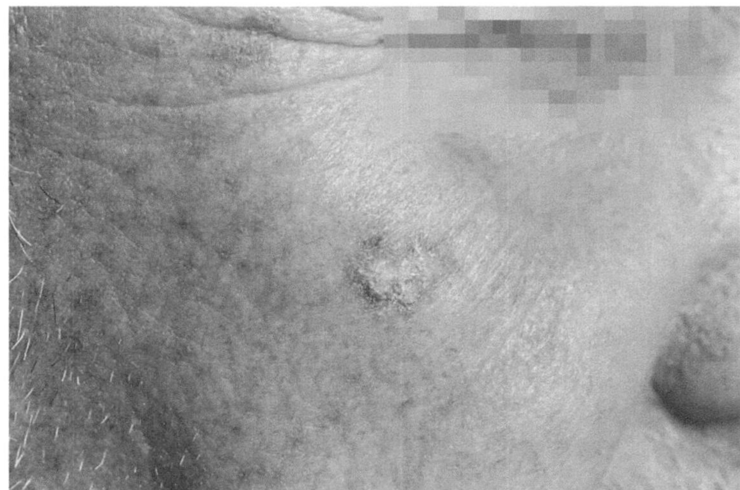

Figure 9.13

Solar keratosis of the cheek in middle-aged woman.

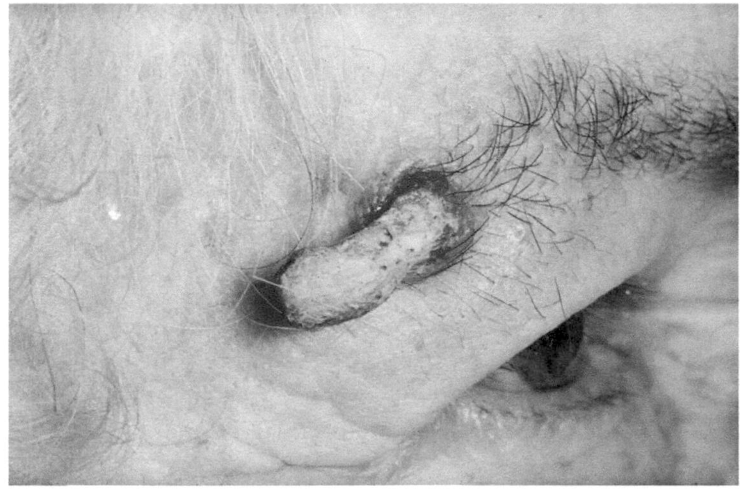

Figure 9.14

Cutaneous horn on basis of solar keratosis.

(Figures 9.15a and 9.15b). The abnormal tissue may be slightly separated from the normal cells and may even give rise to a Darier-like picture.[20]

There is usually an inflammatory cell infiltrate beneath the affected epidermis and in a few cases the infiltrate is band-like and accompanied by basal liquefactive degenerative change giving a lichen planus-like or 'lichenoid' histological picture.[21]

Although solar UVR exposure is the pre-eminent cause of SK, numerous other agencies can also cause keratoses including chronic heat exposure (infrared), X-irradiation, chronic arsenic ingestion, chronic exposure to tar and tar products and some kinds of human papilloma virus infection. In addition, patients who are immunosuppressed either from disease or as part of a therapeutic regimen are prone to the development of large

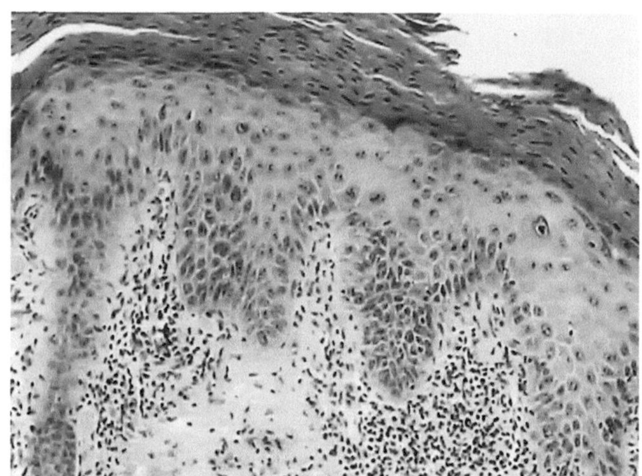

Figure 9.15a

Irregularly thickened epidermis with parakeratosis in solar keratosis. The epidermal cells are larger than normal, and irregular in size and shape (dysplastic) (hematoxylin and eosin × 150).

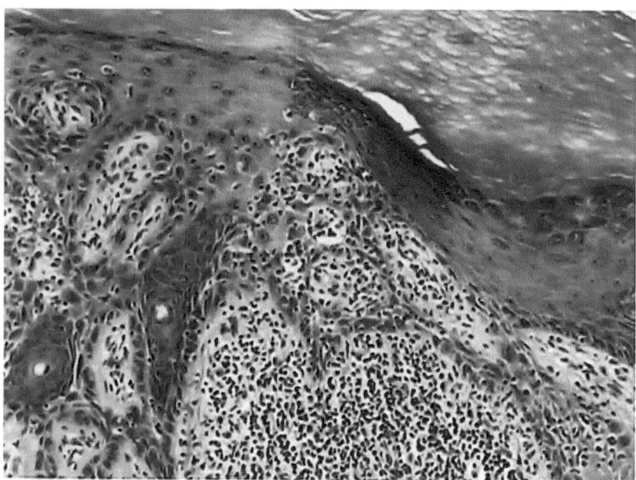

Figure 9.15b

Solar keratosis. The dysplastic epidermis is in marked contrast to the normal epidermis nearby (hematoxylin and eosin × 150).

numbers of SKs. Patients who have received transplants and are on immunosuppressive agents such as ciclosporine or tacrolimus are notoriously at risk – developing more and more SK lesions on sun-exposed sites the longer they have been on the drugs.[22] Patients with HIV disease are often profoundly immunosuppressed and are susceptible to various forms of NMSC, including solar keratoses.

Treatment

It must be borne in mind that SKs signify significant solar damage and should be thought of as the tip of the dysplastic iceberg with the bulk of the epidermal damage as yet undeclared. It must also be remembered that there is very little danger from the individual lesion and the main reason for treatment is cosmetic or for convenience. Only if a lesion enlarges, ulcerates or becomes inflamed is there reason for concern and a determined attempt at ablation.

The large and thick lesions over which there is some doubt need to be formally excised. Smaller palpable SKs are satisfactorily removed by curettage and cautery. Many dermatologists employ cryotherapy with liquid nitrogen when there are multiple small lesions. This is not my favored approach as the technique is always painful and is not as effective as surgical removal. It also has the disadvantage of not yielding a histological answer to the question of diagnosis. When there are multiple lesions it may be best to use chemotherapy with 5% 5-fluorouracil ointment, 3% diclofenac ointment or 5% imiquimod cream. Photodynamic therapy with 5-aminolevulinic acid (or a derivative) is also a satisfactory way of handling these lesions.

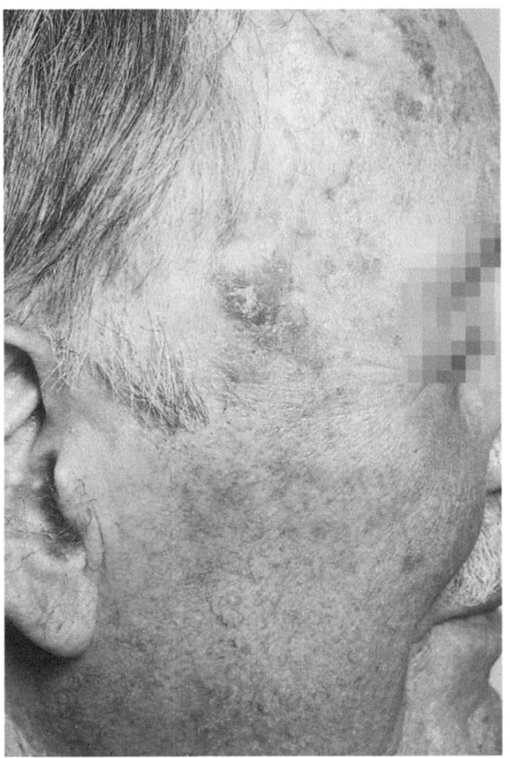

Figure 9.16

This man has a scaling red patch on the right temple that was diagnosed as a solar keratosis but turned out to be a patch of Bowen's disease.

Intraepidermal epithelioma (Bowen's disease)

These are biologically similar to SKs but clinically they tend to be larger and thicker. They sometimes look psoriasiform (Figure 9.16). They occur more often on the trunk and limbs (legs in particular) than do SKs. Intraepidermal epithelioma also occurs on the penis as erythroplasia of Queyrat and on the vulva. Histologically the whole thickness of the epidermis is involved and the affected keratinocytes are even more bizarre than in SK (Figure 9.17).

Treatment is as for SK.

Keratoacanthoma (molluscum sebaceum, KA)

These lesions occur mainly on the face but also on the upper limbs and trunk and show epidermal dysplasia but their exact relationship to malignant and premalignant epidermal lesions is as yet inadequately understood. It seems that there

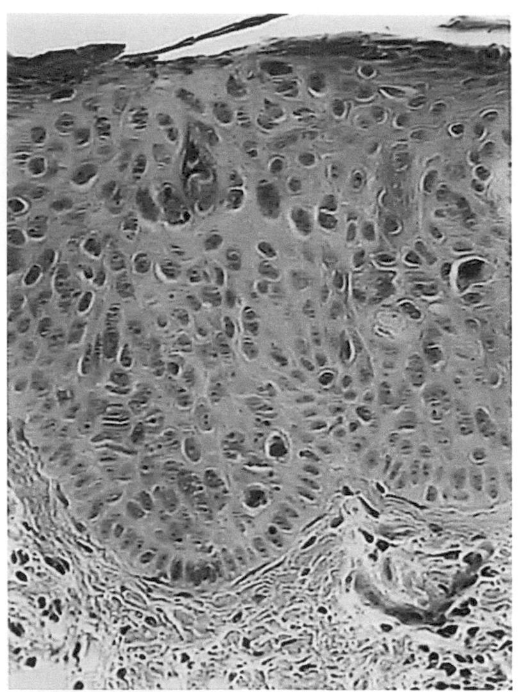

Figure 9.17

Pathology of Bowen's disease. Note the marked dysplasia and epidermal thickening (hematoxylin and eosin × 250).

is a sudden massive stimulus to follicular growth leading to a tumor with the overall architecture of a follicle, which after a while suddenly stops.

Clinical features

Characteristically a rapidly growing warty lesion appears with perpendicular walls, a 'crateriform appearance' and a central horny plug. The KA grows rapidly for up to 6 weeks reaching a maximum of 2–3 cm in diameter. It then remains the same size for a few weeks before regressing over a period of a few weeks or at the most 6 months. Spontaneous regression is often accompanied by unpleasant scarring.

Pathology

There is an invaginated cup-shaped area of epidermal thickening with a central horny plug – so that the whole lesion resembles an enormous distorted follicle. At the sides of the lesion there may be other follicles which show a lesser degree of hypertrophy. There is slight cellular atypia at the margins and an increased number of mitoses. There are also areas of premature keratinization which appear more intensely eosinophilic. It is not easy to distinguish a KA from a well-differentiated SCC histologically – the overall architecture, the degree of dysplasia and the clinical history must all be taken into account.

Squamous cell carcinoma (squamous cell epithelioma, SCC)

Chronic sun exposure is the commonest cause of SCC but in addition SCC may occur from chronic heat injury,[23] at the site of previous radiotherapy, at the margins of ulcers and fistulae, in the scars from lupus vulgaris and chronic discoid lupus erythematosus and other clinically inflamed skin disorders. Chronic arsenic poisoning and exposure to tars and tar products are other well-known causes of SCC. SCC occur much more frequently in the immunosuppressed no matter whether the immunosupppression is 'spontaneous' as in HIV disease or induced therapeutically as in transplant patients. SCC and other forms of NMSC and/or melanoma are

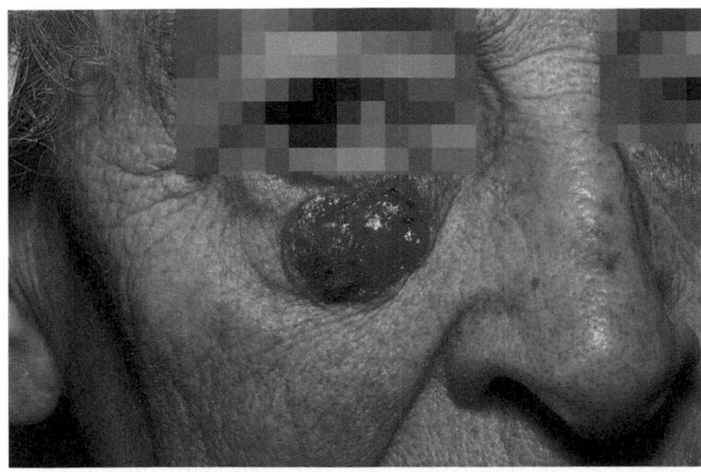

Figure 9.18

Squamous cell carcinoma forming an eroded protuberant nodule affecting the lower eyelid.

also the inevitable results of xeroderma pigmentosum.[24] This is a group of disorders characterized by an inherited defect in one of the enzymes responsible for DNA repair after UVR exposure. The DNA mutations that are 'allowed to remain' by the genetically determined repair deficiency give rise to skin cancers of one sort or another and a premature death from their dissemination.[25]

Clinical appearance

SCC usually present as ulcerated plaques or nodules. There is often a thickened rolled margin but this is not a consistent feature (Figure 9.18). Very indolent lesions can present as cutaneous horns arising from pink slightly thickened plaques. Sometimes they resemble keratoacanthomata and then are difficult to distinguish from these lesions – both clinically and histologically.

Pathology

There are areas of irregularly thickened epidermis which need to be distinguished from the thickening found in benign disorders such as hypertrophic lichen planus or at the edge of chronic ulcers and fistulae (pseudoepitheliomatous hyperplasia). The epidermis shows a variable degree of nuclear atypia and lack of polarization. In some areas there are attempts at keratinization resulting in the formation of horny foci (or horn pearls) (Figure 9.19) and individual dyskeratotic cells.

Treatment and prognosis

In most cases there is a low potential for metastasis. The genitalia, the lips and the ears have the worst reputations for metastatic spread. Surgical excision, microsurgery, photodynamic therapy and laser ablation (e.g. with the CO_2 laser) are the mainstays of treatment.[25] The particular modality used is of course dependent on the size, the site and the aggressiveness of the lesion as well as the health and wishes of the patient. The overall prognosis depends on the site, the stage of the disease and the mode of treatment.[26,27]

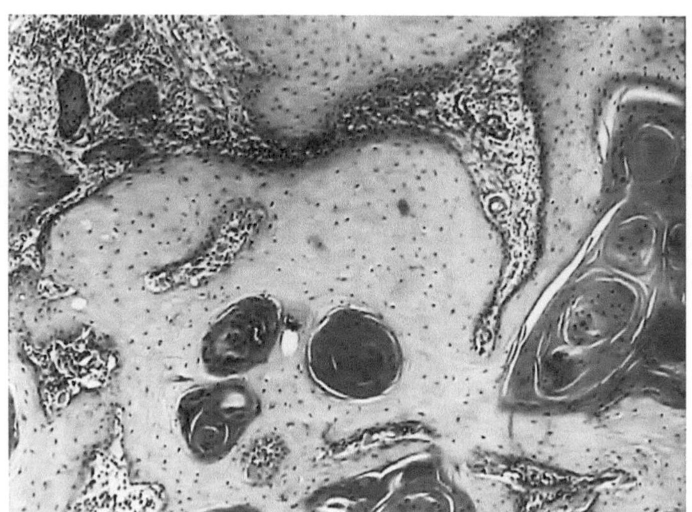

Figure 9.19

There are large irregular masses of dysplastic epidermal tissue containing 'horn pearls' typical of squamous cell carcinoma (hematoxylin and eosin × 150).

Epidermoid cysts

These horn-filled epidermis-lined cavities are common over the face – particularly around the ears and on the forehead. They often 'leak' and become inflamed. Milia are tiny epidermoid cysts that develop high in the dermis following subepidermal blistering and for no known reason.

Pilar cysts (trichilemmal cysts)

These are cysts formed from a part of the hair follicle epithelium. They produce a special type of horn by a specialized process of keratinization (trichilemmal keratinization). Pilar cysts are most common on the scalp and are more common in women. They are not infrequently multiple and are inherited in a dominant fashion. The lining epithelium is sometimes thickened – and rarely gives rise to a squamous cell epithelioma.

Steatocystoma (sebocystoma) multiplex

These uncommon cysts are multiple and generalized. They are lined by sebaceous gland epithelium (and sometimes other follicular elements) and may contain pure sebum. The condition is inherited as a dominant characteristic.

Dermoid cysts

Dermoid cysts are developmental anomalies in which there may be a mixture of epithelia and their products. They are uncommon but are sometimes found on the head and neck.

Melanocytic neoplasms and hamartoma

Melanocytic nevi (moles, nevus cell nevi)

Everyone has a few of these common lesions which probably originate from a faulty sequence of events in the embryonic migration of cells (destined to become melanocytes) from the neural crest to the dermis. They are uncommon in ethnic types with heavily pigmented skin.

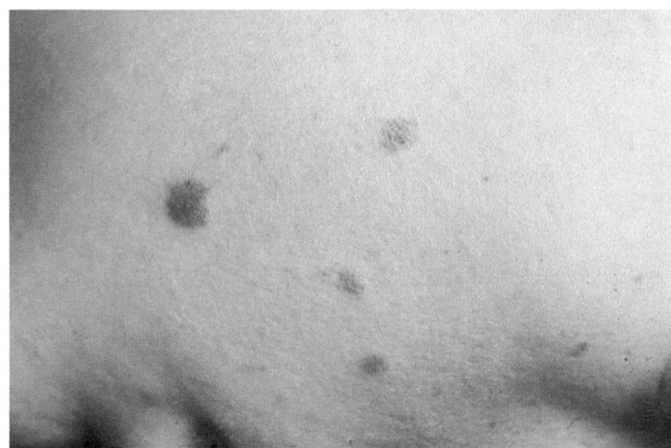

Figure 9.20

Nevus near corner of mouth – a common site.

Some nevi are present at birth or shortly after and these are known as congenital nevi. These latter tend to be larger than acquired nevi and have a bad reputation for giving rise to malignant melanomata. Acquired nevi or nevi that begin to appear in childhood tend to increase in number after sun exposure.

Nevi have an immense range of clinical expression. They vary in size from the tiny (1–2 mm) to the enormous, covering a significant area of the body surface – these giant nevi are often found around the shoulder or pelvic girdles. The color of nevi ranges from the light brown to black or pink and sometimes they are hardly melanized at all. On the face nevi tend to occur around the nasolabial folds and around the mouth (Figure 9.20) and to be only lightly pigmented. Such moles often sprout hair and occasionally become inflamed. They often seem to become more prominent in the elderly – possibly because of degenerate changes which include fatty change, fibrosis and calcification.

Blue nevus

This is a variety of mole which often occurs on the face and scalp. Such lesions appear blue because of the depth of the nevus cells within the skin and the aggregrates of pigment they produce. Red is differentially absorbed from the light reflected back from the pigment, making it look blue – the so-called 'Tyndall effect'.

Nevus of Ota

This is a variety of blue nevus that occurs in Asian peoples, particularly the Japanese. It is very rare in Caucasians and in black-skinned individuals. The nevus is flat, slate-gray or bluish-gray in color and occurs around the eye and on the side of the face and may affect the sclera. The nevus of Ito is similar but occurs around the base of the neck and the shoulders (Figure 9.20a). Both of these congenital lesions are similar in appearance to the Mongolian spot.

Pathology

Nevi contain variously sized aggregates of 'nevus cells'. These aggregrates or 'theques' occur at the dermoepidermal junction in 'young' nevi during their proliferative phase (Figure 9.21). When this is the predominant pattern, they are known as junctional nevi. When the

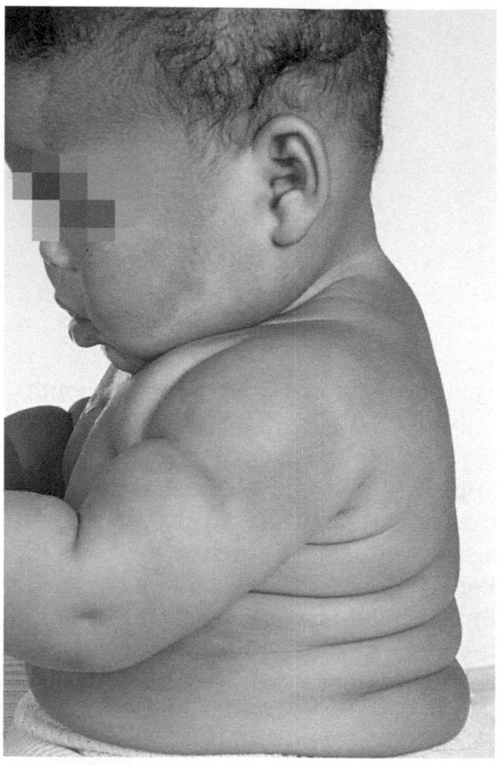

Figure 9.20a

Nevus of Ito affecting face and shoulder.

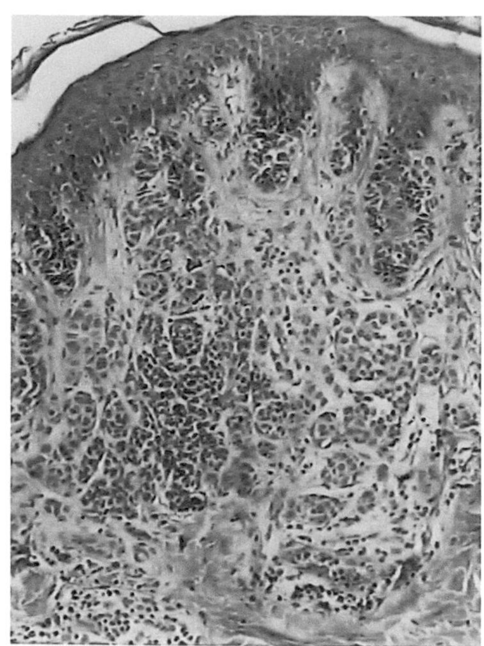

Figure 9.21

Histological picture of compound nevus. 'Buds or nests' of nevus cells can be seen at the dermoepidermal junction as well as aggregates of nevus cells in the dermis (hematoxylin and eosin × 150).

theques occur in the mid-dermis alongside junctional theques, the nevus is known as compound nevus, and when no junctional theques are present, the lesion is known as a dermal cellular nevus. Nevus cells vary greatly in size and shape. They may be small and lymphocyte-like, larger and epithelial-like or spindle-shaped (simulating neural tissue). These latter are characteristic of blue nevi. Giant cells are also quite common in nevi.

Juvenile melanoma

These uncommon and odd nevi occur in children and adolescents predominantly. They are red or pink intracutaneous papules, nodules or plaques, often with a 'peau d'orange' surface, which appear on the face and upper trunk during childhood.

Pathology

Characteristically there is considerable junctional activity and the nevus cells are large, often bizarre and show increased mitotic activity. The histological appearance may resemble malignant melanoma and great care must be taken to distinguish the two kinds of lesion.

Dysplastic nevus

The dysplastic nevus syndrome refers to an uncommon dominantly inherited disorder in which there are multiple odd-looking moles with some of the physical signs of malignant melanoma (MM). They also have an atypical histological appearance with some similarities to MM. The term dysplastic nevus is also applied to individual moles with these characteristics and this has been the cause of considerable contention. There is a much greater risk of dysplastic nevi transforming to MM than ordinary moles.[28]

Fibrous papules of the nose

This is an uncommon benign pink papular lesion occurring on the nose which contains large irregular cells that may be nevocytic in origin.

Birt–Hogg–Dubé syndrome

This is a rare dominantly inherited disorder in which multiple firm dome-shaped papules appear in adults over the head and neck. Histologically, they appear to be fibrofolliculomas. They are associated with lung cysts and renal tumors.[29]

Malignant melanoma

Malignant melanoma (MM) is a malignant neoplasm of epidermal melanocytes. It has shown an increase in incidence worldwide over the past 50 years and has assumed a major importance in public health planning. The incidence rose from 13.5 to 40.0 per 100 000 population per annum in the USA in men aged 35–64 in the 30 years 1969–1999.[30] In Scotland the incidence rose from 3.5 to 10.6 per 100 000 per annum between 1979 and 1998 in men.[31] The greatest increase in incidence appears to be in older men in the head and neck region.

The bulk of the data that have cumulated concerning the cause of the disease and the reason for the increase in incidence point to exposure to solar UVR as being the main agency responsible. In particular, short bursts of intense sun exposure in childhood are thought to be especially dangerous (see Chapter 7). Fair-complexioned and especially red-haired individuals, who do not tan after sun exposure (type I–II subjects, see Chapter 7), are especially at risk. In addition there are genetic and familial susceptibilities unrelated to skin pigmentation.

The 'epidemic' of melanoma, the difficulties in distinguishing some benign moles or seborrheic warts from MM and their potential for lethality despite relatively trivial clinical appearance has generated considerable alarm in the community. These factors have also stimulated an enormous amount of research in all aspects of melanoma to which it is impossible to do justice in this brief summary and the reader is referred to reference 32.

Clinical features

MM are of several distinct types:

1. lentigo maligna LM (LMMM)
2. superficial spreading MM (SSMM)
3. nodular MM (NMM) and
4. acral lentiginous MM (ALMM).

Any pigmented lesion that becomes darker and/or variegate in color and enlarges with an irregular margin must be suspected of being an MM (Figure 9.22).

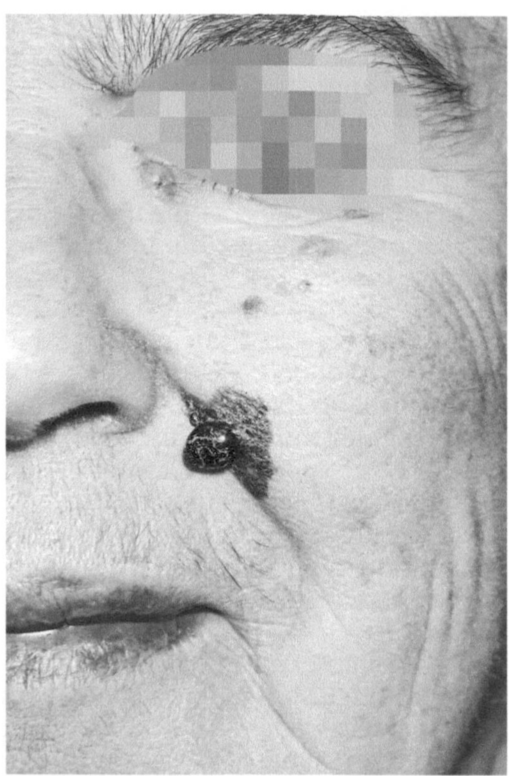

Figure 9.22

Nodular melanoma in late middle-aged woman. The lesion had become increasingly pigmented and enlarged over the previous 3 months.

Approximately 50% of MM arise from a pre-existing nevus. The so-called 'ABCD' rule should help in identifying suspicious lesions, where A = asymmetry, B = irregular border, C = irregular color, and D =>1 cm in diameter. Additionally, surface crusting or oozing, inflammation and itching are other changes that suggest MM. Recent changes in size, color and shape are the core pointers to MM. However, it must be emphasized that even the smartest and most experienced dermatologists sometimes 'get it wrong'. There have been several studies testing the diagnostic acumen of experienced dermatologists for pigmented lesions and it seems more than a 75% accuracy rate is exceptional.[33]

Lentigo maligna (Hutchinson's malignant freckle, LM)

This may be regarded as 'melanoma in situ' in which the abnormal melanocytes stay confined to the epidermis and don't spread outside the lesion. LM characteristically occurs as a slowly enlarging pigmented patch on the face of middle-aged or elderly individuals who show the changes of photodamage (Figure 9.23). Often there is a mixture of shades of brown pigmentation (variegation) which helps distinguish LM from senile lentigo or seborrheic wart. After a variable period a pigmented nodule may arise from LM which must be suspected of being a melanoma (LMMM), which then behaves like a nodular melanoma arising elsewhere.

Pathology

Abnormal melanocytes populate the base of the epidermis and permeate the epidermis. There are prominent pigment deposits in the upper dermis.

Superficial spreading MM

This is the less aggressive type of MM and is thought to be in the 'horizontal growth phase' so that it spreads laterally rather than vertically into deeper tissues. Clinically, SSMM is macular or only just palpable.

Pathology

There are many 'nests' of abnormal melanocytes at the dermoepidermal

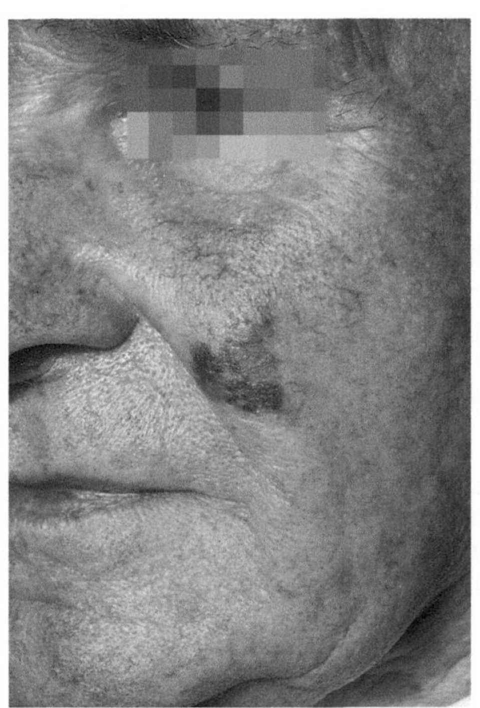

Figure 9.23

Lentigo maligna. This macular lesion increased in size and developed increasing pigmented patches in it over the previous year.

junction and abnormal melanocytic cells in the basal layer as well as permeating the substance of the dermis.

Nodular melanoma (NM)

This form of MM is in the 'vertical growth phase' with groups of abnormal melanocytes extending into the dermis and beyond – the deeper the spread of melanoma tissue, the worse the prognosis. Clinically, NM is a raised nodule or tumor which is irregularly shaped and irregularly pigmented (Figure 9.24). Later in the disease the nodule tends to erode and the surrounding skin may become pigmented and develop satellite nodules. At this stage metastatic spread to regional lymph nodes and later distant nodes occurs as well as spread to the liver, lungs, brain, etc.

Pathology

There is a mass of proliferating abnormal melanocytes at the dermoepidermal junction as well as large aggregates of melanoma cells in the depths of the dermis. Deposits of pigment and a dense inflammatory cell infiltrate are also present. Areas of tumor regression are also seen in many cases.

Acral lentiginous melanoma

This type of melanoma, seen in non-Caucasian subjects, occurs subungually in the fingers and toes and on the palmoplantar skin of the hands and feet. These lesions tend to metastasize early and overall have a poor prognosis.

Prognosis and treatment

The prognosis depends on the depth of invasion of melanoma tissue. The depth of invasion is measured in millimeters from the epidermal granular layer to the deepest level of invasion by the melanoma and is known as the Breslow thickness.[34] The 'Clark level' is a more qualitative evaluation describing the anatomical zone to which the invasion has reached. Other histological features such as mitotic activity, inflammation, involvement of blood vessels, do not appear to give the same degree of accuracy with regard to prognosis.

The definitive treatment is surgical excision – width of the margin being dependent on the Breslow measurement.

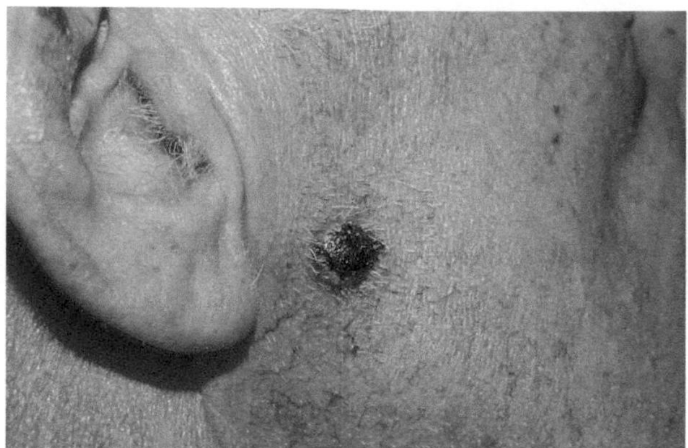

Figure 9.24

Nodular melanoma in preauricular region of elderly man. The lesion had become darker and enlarged in the previous 4 months.

For lesions of 0.5 mm Breslow thickness a margin of 1.0 cm is given with expectation of 95% 5-year survival. For a depth of 1–2 mm a margin of 1–2 cm is given with an expectation of 80–90% 5-year survival. For a depth of 4 mm a 2–3 cm margin is needed with a 5-year life expectancy of 50%.

With lymph node involvement the prognosis becomes very much worse. 'Sentinel node' biopsy is a surgical procedure designed to determine if the main draining lymph node is involved, with initiation of treatment with interferon or other systemic measures if melanoma deposits are found.

Benign lesions and hamartomata of blood vessels

Port wine stains (nevus flammeus)

Flat, dark red or crimson patches often occuring in the distribution of the sensory innervation of the fifth nerve are extremely common and can be unpleasant cosmetically (Figure 9.25). They are unremarkable histologically and all that can be seen is a slight increase in the number of mature but dilated capillaries in the upper dermis. When the patches are extensive and occur in the territory of the ophthalmic branch of the fifth cranial nerve, there may also be an intracranial vascular anomaly which may result in epilepsy or other neurological disturbance. This congenital 'neurocutaneous' disorder is known as the Sturge–Weber syndrome. Port wine stains do not tend to disappear spontaneously although an individual lesion may develop normally colored patches of skin within its confines. In fact these lesions rather than disappearing with the increasing age of the patient may become more prominent by developing hypertrophic and even warty papillomatous areas.

Treatment

The treatment of choice is with lasers, but the age at which treatment is undertaken and the choice of laser depends on the operator.[36] In general the results are excellent.[35] It is of considerable help to the patients to receive adequate advice concerning cosmetic camouflage for any remaining visible birthmark.

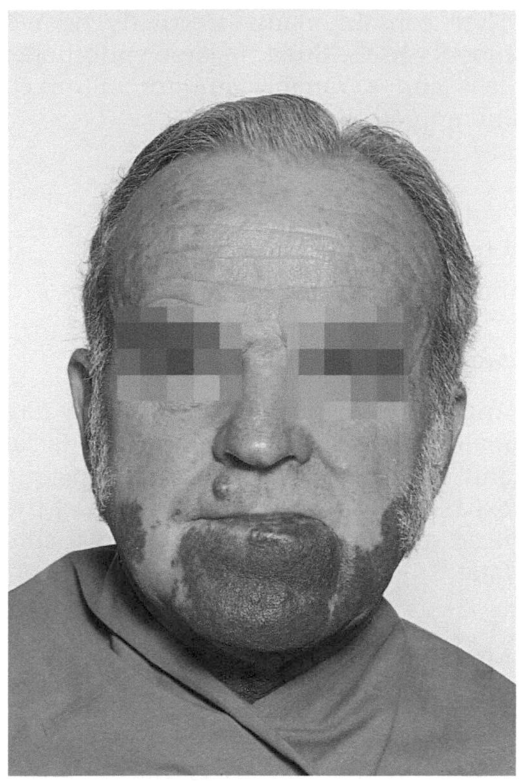

Figure 9.25

Port wine stain affecting chin.

Spider nevus

This lesion mostly occurs on the face and upper limbs. It consists of a central red spot with radiating legs. It is usually an unexplained anomaly but when there are many, liver disease may be present. Sometimes a few lesions appear in pregnancy.

Strawberry nevus (capillary hemangioma)

These lesions are lobulated, raised and bright-red. They vary in size and seem to have an intrinsic growth cycle of their own. In the main they make their appearance in the first few months of life, enlarge during early childhood and then regress in late childhood and the early teens. Rarely they enlarge with frightening rapidity and reach alarming proportions. Giant lesions are sometimes associated with a thrombocytopenia, by virtue of their sequestration of platelets. Some lesions are not 'pure strawberry' but may contain more mature blood vessel elements as well, and then the lesion looks variegate and often bluish in areas. Large lesions not infrequently become traumatized and may ulcerate. In these circumstances they may give rise to troublesome bleeding.

Pathology

These lesions consist of agglomerates of endothelial cells amongst which are vascular channels.

Treatment

This should be resisted unless there is evidence that natural remission is not taking place or there is some pressing medical reason. It has been shown that large lesions diminish in size with systemic corticosteroids and this treatment has proved life-saving at times when there is persistent bleeding due to thrombocytopenia. Injections of gamma interferon have also been reported to be successful. Our as-yet unreported observations in two patients have shown that topical imiquimod used three times per week greatly reduces the size of the lesions after some months. (Patel and Marks–to be published)

Cavernous hemangioma

These are soft bluish tumors that are composed histologically of thick-walled venous channels. Smaller compressible blue swellings are often seen on the lips of elderly individuals. They are generally asymptomatic and are mostly noticed incidentally. The term 'venous lake' is used for these lesions and they probably represent venous dilatations rather than neoplasms.

Pyogenic granuloma

This common lesion is a rapidly appearing red nodule with a moist surface. It may occur in many different sites but frequently arises near the lips or nostrils. Its etiology is unknown and it may be 'reactive' rather than neoplastic.

Pathology

There is a characteristic change in the connective tissue which is edematous and homogenized. Amidst this curious dermal connective tissue are found numerous thin-walled vascular channels and a variable amount of mixed inflammatory cells.

Treatment

The lesions spontaneously regress after a variable period but as they are unsightly or 'get in the way' patients appreciate their removal by curettage and cautery.

Pseudopyogenic granuloma[36,37]

These rare lesions occur as mauve or bluish irregular plaques and nodules on the ears of women. Their natural history is gradually to enlarge, but they are in general asymptomatic.

They contain many irregularly dilated blood vessels, lined by large endothelial cells and a variable amount of mixed inflammatory cells.

Malignant tumors of endothelium

Angioendothelioma

Angioendothelioma is luckily a very rare malignant endothelial tumor of facial and scalp skin in which a red plaque expands to affect most of the skin of the head and neck. It is almost invariably fatal.[38]

Merkel cell tumors

These are quite rare malignant tumors that arise from the neuroendocrine system in the skin. They mostly affect the sun-exposed skin of the elderly and have a significant potential to metastasize. They invade lymphatic channels early on and this fact must be taken into consideration when planning treatment.[39]

References

1. Staples MP, Elwood M, Burton RC et al. Non-melanoma skin cancer in Australia: the 2002 national survey and trend since 1985. Med J Austr 2006; 184: 6–10.
2. Helwig EB. Inverted follicular keratosis. In: Seminar on the Skin; Neoplasms and Dermatoses. Proceedings 20th seminar, American Society of Clinical Pathologists. Int Congress of Clin Path, Washington, DC: Am Soc Clin Path.
3. Sim-Davis D, Marks R, Wilson-Jones E. The inverted follicular keratosis. A surprising

variant of seborrheic wart. Acta Derm Venereol 1976; 56: 337–44.

4. Munoz-Perez MA, Garcia-Hernandez MJ, Rios JJ, Camacho F. Sebaceous naevi: a clinicopathologic study. J Eur Acad Dermatol Venereol 2002; 16: 319–24.
5. Lee SH, Rogers M. Inflammatory linear verrucous epidermal naevi: a review of 23 cases. Australas J Dermatol 2001; 42: 252–6.
6. Hofer T. Does inflammatory linear verrucous epidermal naevus represent a segmental type 1/type 2 mosaic of psoriasis? Dermatology 2006; 212: 103–7.
7. Happle R, Koopman RJ. Becker naevus syndrome. Am J Med Genet 1997; 68: 357–61.
8. Sugarman JL. Epidermal nevus Syndromes. Semin Cutan Med Surg 2004; 23: 145–57.
9. Nissen B, Marks R. Eruptive syringoma, a clinicopathological study of thirty-five patients. Br J Dermatol Suppl 1974; 10: 20.
10. Lan MY, Lan MC, Ho CY et al. Pilomatricoma of the head and neck: a retrospective review of 179 cases. Arch Otolaryngol Head Neck Surg 2003; 129: 1237–30.
11. Harper PS. Calcifying epithelioma of Malherbe. Association with myotonic muscular dystrophy. Arch Dermatol 1972; 106: 41–4.
12. Madan V, Hoban P, Strange RC et al. Genetics and risk factors for basal cell carcinoma. Br J Derm 2006;154(Suppl 1): 5–7.
13. Rowe DE, Carroll RJ, Day CL Jr. Moh's surgery is the treatment of choice for recurrent (previously treated) basal cell carcinoma. J Dermatol Surg Oncol 1989; 15: 424–13.
14. Brown SB. The role of light in the treatment of non-melanoma skin cancer using methyl aminolaevulinate. J Derm Treat 2003; 14(Suppl 3): 11–14.
15. Ionescu DN, Arida M, Jukic DM. Metastatic basal cell carcinoma: four case reports, literature and immunohistochemical evaluation. Arch Pathol Lab Med 2006; 130: 45–51.
16. Marks R, Ponsford MW, Selwood TS et al. Non-melanotic skin cancer and solar keratoses in Victoria. Med J Austral 1983; 2: 619–22.
17. Harvey I, Frankel S, Marks R et al. Non melanoma skin cancer and solar keratoses. I. Methods and descriptive results of the South Wales Cancer Study. Br J Cancer 1996; 74: 1302–7.
18. Memon AA, Tomenson JA, Bothwell J, Friedmann PS. Prevalence of solar damage and actinic keratosis in a Merseyside population. Br J Dermatol 2000; 144: 1154–9.
19. Marks R, Rennie G, Selwood TS. Malignant transformation of solar keratoses to squamous cell carcinoma. Lancet 1988; I: 795–7.
20. Lever L, Marks R. The significance of the Darier-like solar keratosis and acantholytic change in preneoplastic lesions of the epidermis. Br J Dermatol 1989; 120: 383–9.
21. Tan CY, Marks R. Lichenoid solar keratoses. Prevalence and immunological findings. J Invest Dermat 1982; 79: 365–7.
22. Veness MJ, Quinn DI, Ong CS et al. Aggressive cutaneous malignancies following cardiothoracic transplantation: the Australian experience. Cancer 1999; 85: 1758–64.
23. Onugbo WI. Epidemiology of skin cancer arisen from the burn scars in Nigerian Ibos Burns 2006;
24. Broughton BC, Cordonnier A, Kleijer WJ et al. Molecular analysis of mutations in DNA polymerase in xeroderma pigmentosum patients. Proc Natl Acad Sci USA 2002; 99: 815–20.
25. Roberts DJ, Cairnduff F. Photodynamic therapy of primary skin cancer: a review. Br J Plast Surg 1995; 48: 360–70.
26. Lewis KG, Weinstock MA. Nonmelanoma skin cancer mortality (1988–2000): the Rhode Island and follow-back study. Arch Dermatol 2004; 140: 837–42.
27. Rowe DE, Carroll DJ, Day CL et al. Prognostic factors for local recurrence, metastasis and survival rates in squamous cell carcinoma of the skin, ear and lip. Implications for treatment modality selection. J Am Dermatol 1992; 26: 976–90.
28. Ferrone CR, Porat L, Panageus KS. Clinicopathological features and risk factors

for multiple primary melanomas. JAMA 2005; 294: 1647–54.

29. Vincent A, Farley M, Chan E et al. Birt–Hogg–Dubé syndrome. A review of the literature and the differential diagnosis of firm facial papules. J Am Acad Dermatol 2003; 49: 698–705.
30. Jemal A, Devesa SS, Hartge P, Tucker MA. Recent trends in melanoma incidence amoung whites in the United States. J Natl Cancer Inst 2001; 93: 678–83.
31. MacKie RM, Bray CA, Hole DJ et al. Incidence of and survival from malignant melanoma in Scotland. Lancet 2002; 360: 587–91.
32. Hölzle E, Kind P, Plewig G et al. Malignant Melanoma Diagnosis and Differential Diagnosis. Stuttgart: Schattauer, 1993.
33. Moricrieff M, Cotton S, Claridge E et al. Spectrophotometric intracutaneous analysis: a new technique for imaging pigmented skin lesions. Br J Dermatol 2002; 146: 448–57.
34. Elder DE, Gimotty PA, Guerry D. Cutaneous melanoma: estimating survival and recurrence risk. Dermatol Ther 2005; 18: 369–85.
35. Railan D, Parlette EC, Uebelhoer NS, Rohrer TE. Laser treatment of vascular lesions. Clin Dermatol 2006; 24: 8–15.
36. Wilson-Jones E, Bleehan SS. Inflammatory angiomatous nodules with abnormal blood vessels occurring about the ears and the scalp. Br J Dermatol 1969; 81: 804.
37. Wilson-Jones E. Malignant angioendothelioma of the skin. Br J Dermatol 1964; 76: 21.
38. Paulsen M. Merkel cell carcinoma of skin: diagnosis and management strategies. Drugs Aging 2005; 22: 210–29.
39. Acebo E, Vidaurrazaga N, Varas C et al. Merkel cell carinoma: a clinical pathological study of 11 cases. J Eur Acad Dermatol Venereol 2005; 19: 546–51.

Infections of facial skin

Bacterial infections of facial skin

Impetigo

This is a common infectious disorder of skin caused in most instances by *Staphylococcus aureus*. In a few cases beta-hemolytic streptococci (*Streptococcus pyogenes*) appear responsible. It is the third most common skin disorder in children. Clinically lesions appear on the face, arms or trunk mainly. Blisters sometimes develop (bullous impetigo) and the lesion develops a characteristic golden yellow crust (Figure 10.1). The disorder is mainly a disease of childhood with maximum incidence aged 2–6 years. It is markedly contagious and spreads rapidly within schools so that affected children ought to be excluded from school while the disease is still active. It was found to increase in prevalence in the Netherlands from 16.5 per 100 in children under the age of 18 to 20.6 per 1000 under the age of 18 between 1987 and 2001.[1] After the acute stage, the disorder 'settles down' to form a spreading pink scaly patch which may be misdiagnosed as eczema, psoriasis or even ringworm.

In humid subtropical areas underprivileged and sometimes immunocompromised children may develop a severe skin infection caused by streptococcus (*Strep. pyogenes*) which has sometimes been called impetigo but is better known as ecthyma. The lesion is erosive or ulcerative and may be followed by acute glomerulonephritis.

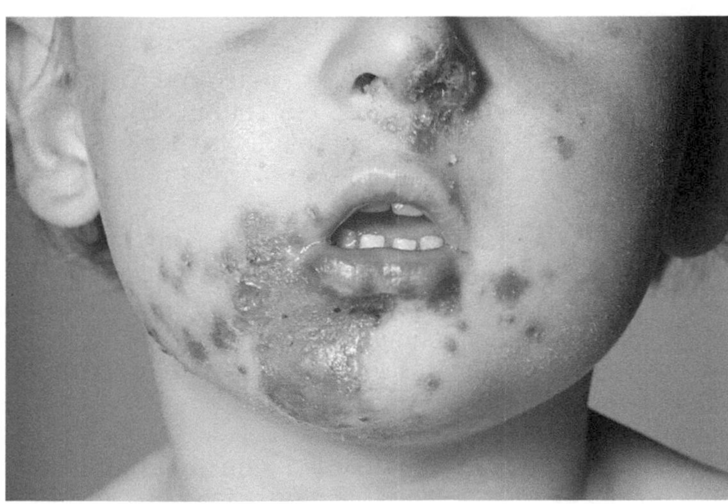

Figure 10.1

There is a patch of impetigo on the jaw in this child.

Treatment

For patients with limited uncomplicated impetigo, topical mupirocin or fusidic acid for 7 days should suffice. One study showed that topical tetracycline was as effective as oral antibiotics.[2] If systemic treatment is required, flucloxacillin or ciprofloxacin are appropriate treatments.

Erysipelas

This is a skin infection caused by the beta-hemolytic group A streptococcus of particular serotype. It affects the skin of the face and lower legs in most cases causing a characteristic rash (Figure 10. 2) and a severe systemic pyrexial illness. The rash is red, edematous and well-defined. Bonnetblanc and Bedane provide an excellent review of the topic.[3] As the condition gradually spreads it causes considerable tissue destruction and unpleasant scarring. There may be hemorrhagic vesiculation at the margins. It starts suddenly and spreads rapidly. It is particularly devastating in the elderly and before the antibiotic era was not infrequently fatal.

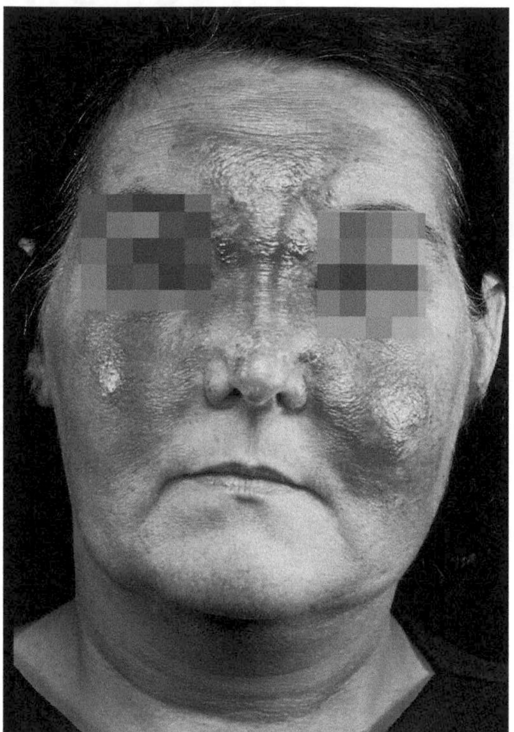

Figure 10.2

Erysipelas. The affected areas are swollen, hot and tender and the patient is usually pyrexial and very unwell.

Treatment

Treatment is with antibiotics and usually penicillin or a macrolide antibiotic is sufficient. The response is usually dramatic.

Boils, carbuncles and sycosis barbae

These are all infections of the facial hair follicles with pyogenic pathogenic bacteria – usually *Staphylococcus aureus*. These disorders have become progressively uncommon with increasing societal hygiene. Boils are red, tender papules or nodules of varying size. Most drain pus after some days. Boils may develop in clusters and often staphylococci can be isolated from nasal swabs in patients with multiple or recurrent boils.

Carbuncles are large lesions that result from the infections of several follicles coalescing into a single large lesion. Such lesions may cause severe systemic upset. The treatment is with the appropriate antibiotics.

Sycosis barbae is a folliculitis of the beard area. The infection appears to affect the superficial parts of the facial hair follicles in men causing papules and papulopustules (Figure 10.3). It is caused at least in part or aggravated by the trauma of shaving. It has to be distinguished from acne and from the condition known as pili recurvati. This latter disorder is seen in the beard hair follicles of black-skinned individuals, on the neck in particular. It is due to the beard hair shafts emerging at odd angles from the skin surface and the cut end growing back into the skin causing multiple small inflammatory papules. The treatment of sycosis barbae is with topical antibiotics (e.g. fusidic acid or mupirocin), antimicrobial washes and disposable razors. On the face it may be mistaken for acute systemic lupus erythematosus or acute allergic contact dermatitis.

Lupus vulgaris

This is a rare chronic infection with the tubercle bacillus, often affecting the face. It causes a slowly spreading granulomatous plaque and cluster of papules. When a glass slide is pressed on these they appear translucent but have a central opaque yellowish brown center – the so-called 'apple-jelly' sign (Figure 10.4). As the condition gradually slowly spreads it causes considerable tissue destruction and unpleasant scarring. Histologically there is granulomatous inflammation but little in the way (if any) of caseation necrosis. It is rare to find the tubercle bacillus in the lesion. The treatment is as for tuberculosis elsewhere with 'triple therapy'.[4]

Tinea faciei and barbae

These are names used to describe dermatophytosis or ringworm infection of facial skin. Although not common the condition is by no means rare and is often misdiagnosed.[5,6] It may be more common in hot humid climates. Any of the ringworm species appear capable of infecting facial skin and the condition

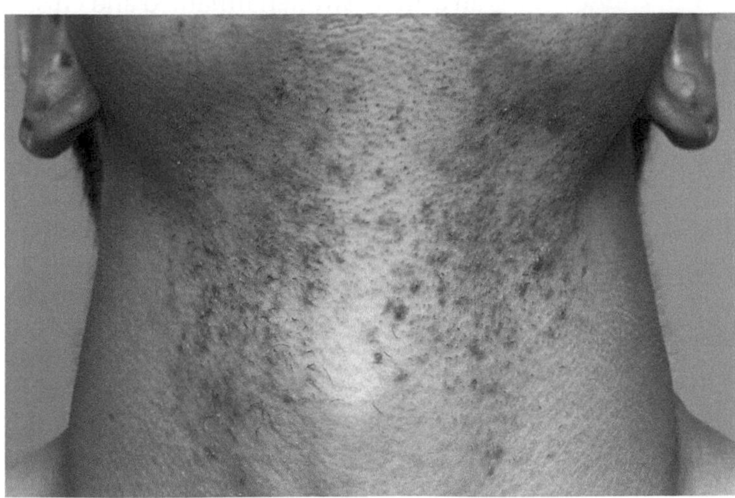

Figure 10.3

Sycosis barbae. There are inflamed papules and papulopustules affecting the follicular orifices on the front of the neck.

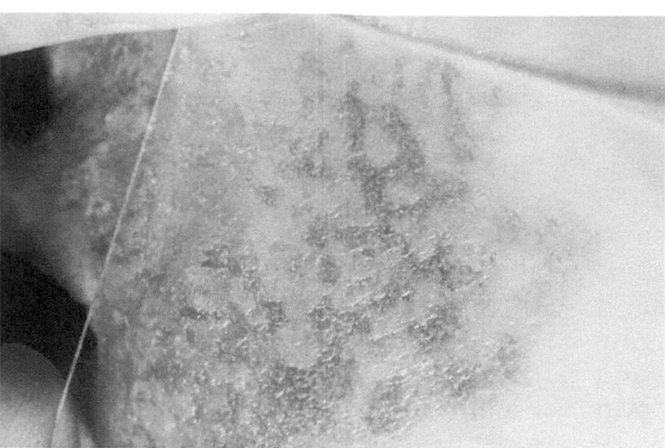

Figure 10.4

Lupus vulgaris. A microscope slide is pressed against the lesion to show the small apple-jelly nodules of granuloma (diascopy) typical of this disorder.

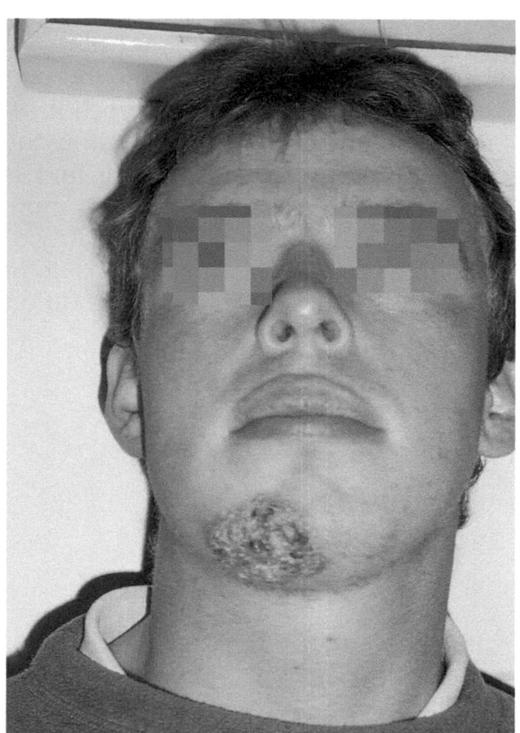

Figure 10.5

Acute inflammatory ringworm of the face.

parades in a variety of uniforms. Nondescript but well-defined scaling pink patches are probably the type of rash most often seen.

Tinea barbae

Tinea barbae refers to the now uncommon disorder of beard follicles in which follicular papules and papulopustules are part of the picture. In some patients there is an acutely swollen inflamed and crusted lesion known as a kerion (Figure 10.5). Children and the immunocompromised are mainly affected by this fungal condition. Ringworm infection is diagnosed by identifying fungal hyphae in scales from the rash either by using the classical KOH method or by taking superficial samples using the skin surface biopsy technique[7] (Figure 10.6). Mycological culture will also reveal the particular species responsible. The condition is often misdiagnosed as eczema[8] and is then treated mistakenly with topical corticosteroids or pimecrolimus or tacrolimus. These anti-inflammatory agents may change

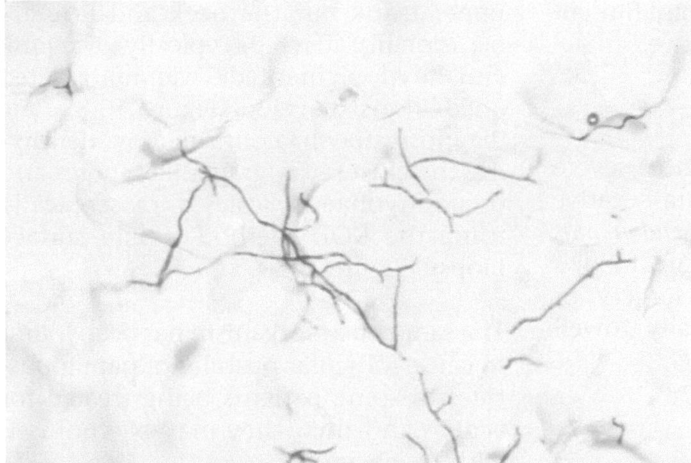

Figure 10.6

Skin surface biopsy from area of ringworm showing fungal hyphae stained by the periodic acid–Schiff reagent (× 45).

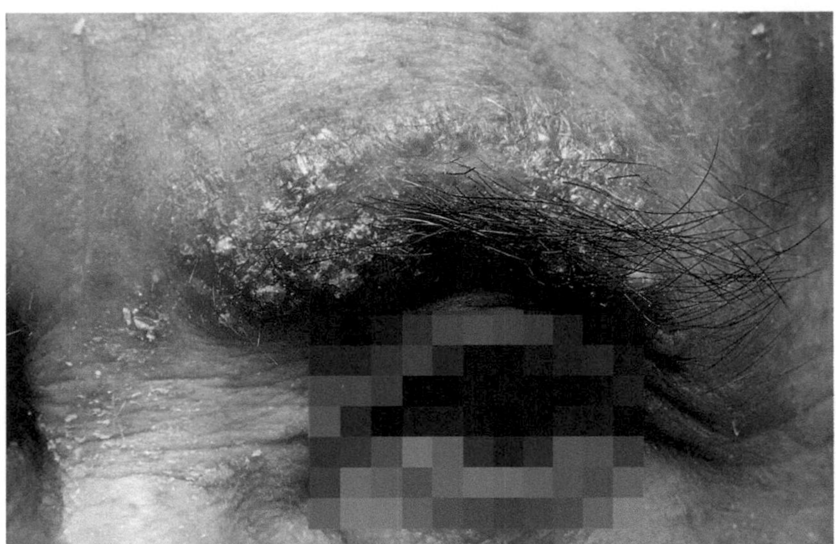

Figure 10.7

Tinea incognito. The usual appearance of ringworm has been altered by the use of topical corticosteroids.

the appearance from that of a typical ringworm-like rash to an unrecognizable disorder – so-called tinea incognito[9] (Figure 10.7).

Treatment

Topical imidazoles such as miconazole or clotrimazole or newer topical agents such as terbinafine are usually sufficient to clear the disorder. Oral terbinafine or itraconazole are reliably effective.

Facial cellulitis

Several reports have appeared of severe facial cellulitis from Gram-negative micro-organisms such as *Pseudomonas aeruginosa*.[10] The cellulitis usually follows dental infections, sinusitis, surgery or trauma. Patients are systemically unwell and have fever.

Pityriasis versicolor

This is a very common mild skin infection with the yeast-like micro-organism *Malassezia furfur* or *Pityrosporum ovale*. This micro-organism is part of the normal follicular flora and only starts to become pathogenic when conditions are favorable to its growth. Hot humid conditions encourage this yeast–like micro-organism as does immunosuppression. Pityriasis versicolor mainly occurs on the upper trunk but the neck and face are occasionally affected. Typically, oval pink and hypopigmented well-marginated 'medallions' develop (Figure 10.8). The diagnosis may be confirmed by identifying the clusters of 'grape-like' spores and pseudohyphae in scales microscopically using the KOH method or skin surface biopsy (Figure 10.9).

The same micro-organism has been found to cause follicular pustules or papulopustules in some patients being treated for acne – and then they may be confused with true acne.

Treatment

Topical imidazoles combined with ketoconazole shampoos are usually adequate but a 10-day course of itraconazole 100 mg daily is thought to be superior by some clinicians. The condition appears to 'hang on' longer than it actually does as the depigmented areas take several

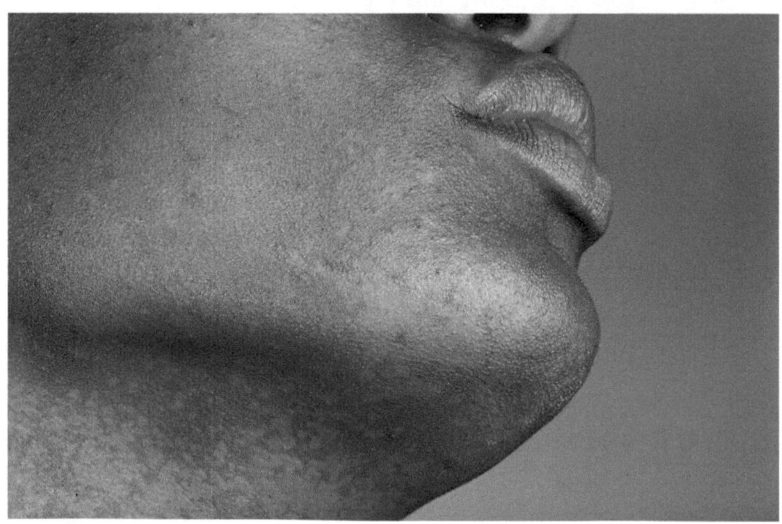

Figure 10.8

Pale round areas on neck and lower face due to pityriasis versicolor.

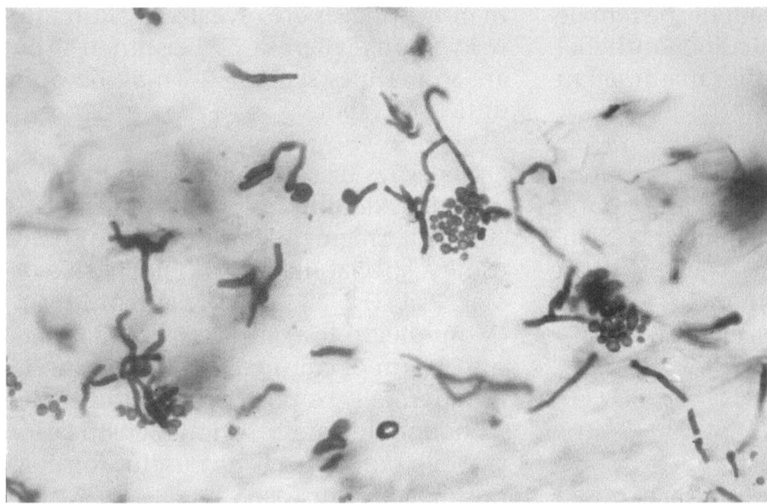

Figure 10.9

Skin surface biopsy from area of pityriasis versicolor showing the typical pseudomycelium and grape-like clusters of spores (periodic acid–Schiff reagent × 45).

months to reach their previous level of pigmentation.

Candidiasis (syn. moniliasis)

Infection with *Candida albicans* of the skin of the face does not usually occur other than as incidental colonization of a pre-existing diseased area (e.g. eczema or angular cheilitis). In angular cheilitis facial and dental changes that occur with aging result in 'overlap' at the lip commissures causing maceration and cracking – ideal soil for candididal superinfections. *Candida albicans* may also cause problems in the immunosuppressed patient resulting in monilial granuloma occurring either in isolation or as part of chronic mucocutaneous candidiasis. Monilial granuloma is not confined to the face as the scalp and skin elsewhere are not infrequently involved. Infants and young children are mostly affected.

Monilial granuloma affects the whole skin thickness and causes a swollen crusted mass with draining sinuses.

Treatment

Initial debridment is often required with subsequent treatment by systemic agents such as itraconazole, amphotericin B and fluconazole.

Leishmaniasis

Cutaneous leishmaniasis is cutaneous infection with the protozoal organism *Leishmania donovani infantum*, *Leishmania major* and *Leishmania tropica*. It occurs in the Gulf States, Turkey, Greece and elsewhere around the Mediterranean littoral as well as in North Africa and in India. It is spread by the sandfly (*Phlebotomus papatasi* in the Old World and *Lutzomyia* in the New World). The condition is a zoonosis with the reservoir being in dogs and other small mammals. The *Leishmania* parasite develops in the gut of the female sandfly and in the reticuloendothelial system or dermis of the mammalian host.

The disorder is seen at all ages but is especially frequent in infants and young children, especially in endemic areas. The incubation period after a bite by an infected sandfly is extremely variable and ranges from just a week or two to up to several months.

Clinical presentation

One or several lesions develop on exposed sites, especially the face, neck and arms. The appearances of the lesion(s) are dependent on the host's resistance and the particular type of *Leishmania* microorganism involved. Generally the lesion is inflamed and 'boil-like', being swollen and a shade of red. The lesion crusts, mostly ulcerates and eventually scars, taking some months for this sequence to occur.

There are also two chronic forms of the disease which do not spontaneously heal – a lupoid form (the recidivans form) in which plaques of coalescing papules resembling lupus vulgaris spread near a scar and a diffuse cutaneous form which spreads involving large areas. The latter is due to *Leishmania aethiopica* in most cases and in both types there is a failure of immune defenses.

Histologically, the picture is that of a diffuse granuloma. Necrosis does occur but is variable and there may be difficulties in distinguishing the condition from tuberculosis and sarcoidosis. The small rounded parasite bodies (amastingotes) in macrophages are revealed by Romanowsky stains (Giemsa or Leishman's) but are sometimes sparse and may be quite difficult to spot.

Other ways of confirming the diagnosis include examining stained smears and culturing fragments or imprints of tissue using a special medium – Nicolle–Novy–MacNeal (NNN). The leishmanin test (Montenegro test) injects a standardized suspension of cultured *Leishmania* species intradermally. A positive reaction in 48–72 hours indicates previous sensitization at some point and is not useful for diagnosing active disease.

Treatment

Local destruction of the lesion by curettage under local anesthetic or freezing with carbon dioxide snow may be tried. Local injection of sodium stibogluconate or meglumine antimoniate on several occasions is also employed. Systemic antimonial drugs or pentamidine isethionate are used for recalcitrant disease.

New World leishmaniasis and visceral leishmaniasis have not been described as they are beyond the scope of this book.

Herpes simplex virus infections

Herpes viruses are ubiquitous large DNA viruses. There are eight viruses in the herpes simplex group but only herpes simplex I, herpes virus II (HSVI and HSVII) and the zoster-varicella virus will be discussed here. The viruses affect the skin and mucosa but have the interesting habit of hibernating in the dorsal nerve root ganglia of sensory nerves.

They have the ability to reactivate and migrate from the ganglia to cause new episodes of disease.

Herpes simplex I (HSVI)

This virus causes common 'cold sores' around the mouth and nose. In a small proportion of cases the infection starts off as a pyrexial gingivostomatitis. This 'primary infection' affects children 1–3 years of age mostly, causing swollen white patches on the oral mucosa which are studded with vesicles and often ulcerate. The condition causes considerable malaise and lasts 1–2 weeks.

The recurrent attacks of 'cold sores' affect some 5–10% of the population but the frequency of the recurrences is extremely variable, many only being troubled once or twice per year. Typically, recurrent attacks present as inflamed patches surmounted by clusters of papulovesicles and vesicles on the lips, around the mouth or elsewhere on the lower face (Figure 10.10). Such lesions are often preceded by pain and/or paresthesiae at the site. Recurrences are precipitated by all manner of stimuli including a rise in body temperature (which is why they tend to appear at the time of an upper respiratory tract infection – 'cold sores'), exposure to the sun, by a reduction in immune defenses for one reason or another and by simpletrauma. The vesicles dry and become crusted and the inflammation subsides within 7–10 days.

Complications

Eczema herpeticum

Patients with atopic eczema are curiously prone to viral infections of the skin and the development of widespread lesions of *H. simplex* after contact with an infected individual is an example of this. Such patients have widespread vesicles with exudation and crusting as well as being pyrexial and systemically unwell.

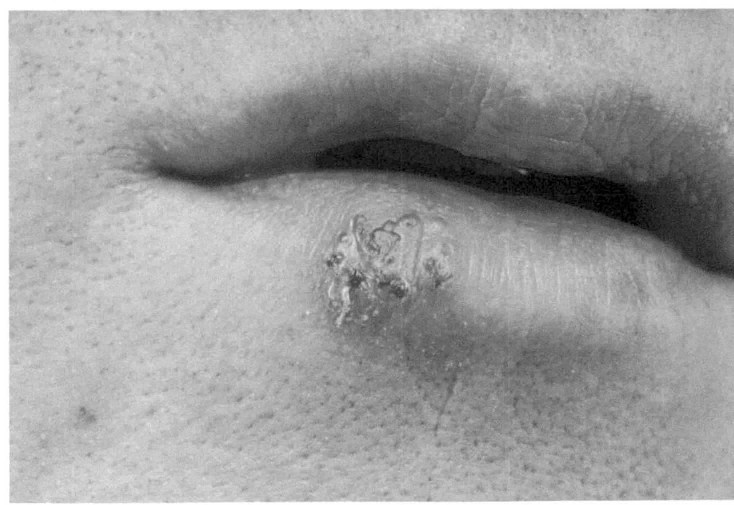

Figure 10.10

Herpes simplex affecting lower lip ('cold sore').

Erythema multiforme
This common eruptive skin disorder seems to be provoked by *H. simplex* in more than half of the patients with the rash. The PCR test has identified *H. simplex* DNA in erythema multiforme lesions[11] but the details of the pathogenesis are obscure.

Keratitis
HSV can cause recurrent painful corneal ulceration.

Herpes simplex II (HSVII – herpes genitalis)

This herpes virus affects the genital mucosae and is spread by sexual contact. Lesions may develop in men on the glans penis, the foreskin as well as the shaft of the penis and occasionally the scrotal skin. In woman lesions may occur over the labia majora or labia minora, and the clitoris and sometimes the cervix. HSVII can also occur elsewhere around the pelvic girdle – particularly the buttocks. Perianal lesions may develop in male homosexuals. As with the HSVI infections, recurrent attacks are often preceded by paresthesiae or pain. Recurrent attacks are extremely common after HSVII infection and are precipitated by the same stimuli as are HSVI infections.

It is interesting to note that genital herpes affects some 55 million people of the USA population, of whom only 20–25% are aware of their condition.[12] The disorder appears to have spread extensively in the Western world and has caused much alarm and despondency in the sexually active segment of the population.

Treatment

Unfortunately there is no curative treatment available for either herpes simplex or genitalis, but there are antiviral drugs that accelerate healing and reduce the severity of the disease. However, for many patients symptomatic measures are all that are needed. These latter include analgesics, topical antimicrobials and mildly astringent lotions when the lesions are exudative and antibiotic or antibiotic/corticosteroid combinations when the lesions are drying and in resolution.

Aciclovir, famciclovir and valaciclovir all interfere with the action of viral DNA polymerase and prevent viral propagation. Valaciclovir is the pro-drug of aciclovir and famciclovir is the pro-drug of penciclovir. Aciclovir given iv 5 mg/kg 8-hourly is the treatment of choice for severe herpes or its complications. It may also be given orally 200 mg five times daily. Oral famciclovir given twice daily (125–500 mg) was found to shorten the time to healing and to reduce the symptoms in recurrent genital herpes in a large placebo-controlled study. Oral twice-daily aciclovir or famciclovir may also be given as a prophylactic measure to prevent recurrences but the efficacy of this seems less than perfect in otherwise normal individuals but may be of particular help to those who are immunocompromised.

Aciclovir cream 5% (Zovirax) may be employed for simple recurrences of herpes simplex or genitalis. It needs to be started at the first symptom and used five times daily to give it the best chance of therapeutic success.

Herpes zoster-varicella

This DNA virus causes chicken pox (varicella) during the initial viremic stage of the infection which will not be described further here. The virus becomes dormant in dorsal root ganglia and herpes zoster (shingles) is the result of reactivation. Zoster is usually, but not necessarily a disorder of the elderly and is more frequent and more severe in the immunosuppressed. Any dorsal root can be affected but thoracic sites are involved in about 60% of cases. Involvement of the trigeminal ganglion with ophthalmic distribution or a maxillary distribution are other quite common manifestations of herpes zoster (Figure 10.11). Herpes zoster usually starts with paresthesiae and pain in the affected area. This is usually followed by the development of swollen erythematous patches along the distribution of the nerve root involved. This is rapidly followed by the appearance of vesicles which successively become purulent, necrotic and crusted. The whole sequence takes 14–28 days on the trunk but longer for ophthalmic zoster. Complications of ophthalmic zoster include uveitis, keratitis and ocular muscle palsies. Zoster of the maxillary division of the trigeminal nerve causes vesicles on the uvula and tonsillar areas in addition to lesions on the cheek. Mandibular zoster causes lesions on the floor of the mouth and the buccal mucosae. Post-herpetic neuralgia (pain persisting more than a month after resolution of the rash) is one of the most common complications. It develops more frequently in the elderly, affecting some 30% of these over the age of 40. The pain may be very disturbing and has both a sharp quality and distorted paresthetic quality. It is more common after trigeminal neuralgia.

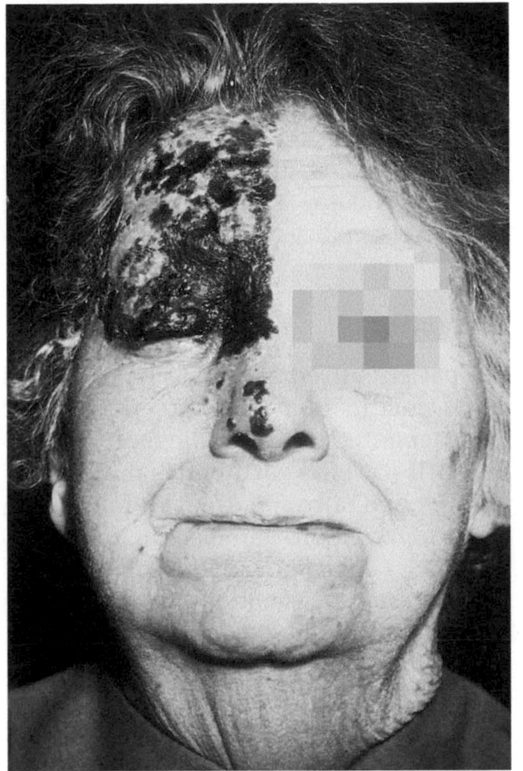

Figure 10.11

Herpes zoster affecting the ophthalmic branch of the fifth nerve (ophthalmic herpes) causing inflammation and crusting around the forehead and peri-ocular region on the affected side.

The development of sparse papulovesicles outside of the affected nerve root is not uncommon and is more often seen in patients who are immunosuppressed.

The Ramsay Hunt syndrome causes sensorineural hearing loss, dizziness and vertigo, impairment of taste and lacrimation. It results from herpes zoster oticus in which the skin of the external auditory meatus is affected as is the soft palate mucosa and occurs alongside facial nerve palsy.

Treatment

All patients need adequate pain control and topical treatment to prevent or counter infection and alleviate discomfort. All patients with ophthalmic zoster require oral antiviral drugs in full dosage such as aciclovir, famciclovir or valaciclovir.[13] Expert ophthalmological assistance should be sought at the first sign of inflammatory disease of the eye.

Viral warts

Viral warts, i.e. benign epidermal tumors caused by infection with one of the human papilloma viruses (HPV), are universal and constitute a major problem in dermatological practice. There are more than 100 serotypes but only a few affect facial skin on any regular basis. The HPV are double-stranded DNA viruses that affect several mammalian species. The commonest clinical types of facial wart are flat warts which appear to be caused by serotypes 3, 10, 28 and 49. Other types may be responsible in the rare condition of epidermodysplasia verruciformis. Flat warts (plane warts) are common in children and young adults (Figure 10.12) and seem to be mainly a problem on the lower face and neck. Filiform warts are also quite common – these annoying often hair-like excrescences are often seen periorificially – around the lips and nostrils.

Warts are very much more prolific in the immunocompromised (Figure 10.12a) – they are, for example, often a problem in patients with HIV disease. They are also more common and in greater numbers in patients with lymphomas – such as Hodgkin's disease. Interestingly they are also more often seen in patients with atopic dermatitis.

All warts spontaneously resolve after some months or years and their resolution is probably the result of an immunological response.

Management

Treatment is rarely required as all these lesions spontaneously resolve – most going within 6 months. If treatment is needed, a salicyclic acid preparation can be used with care – treating only the warts and not the surrounding skin to avoid severe inflammation. Other non-invasive treatments that can be used include diphencyprone sensitization[14] or use of 5% imiquimod cream.[15]

Molluscum contagiosum

Molluscum contagiosum (MC) is due to infection with a large DNA virus that is a member of the pox virus group. It causes small umbilicated 1–3 mm diameter tumors from which may be expressed a semi-solid cheesey core (Figure 10.13). They are most common in children and are frequently seen on the face. As with warts they are sometimes a sign of

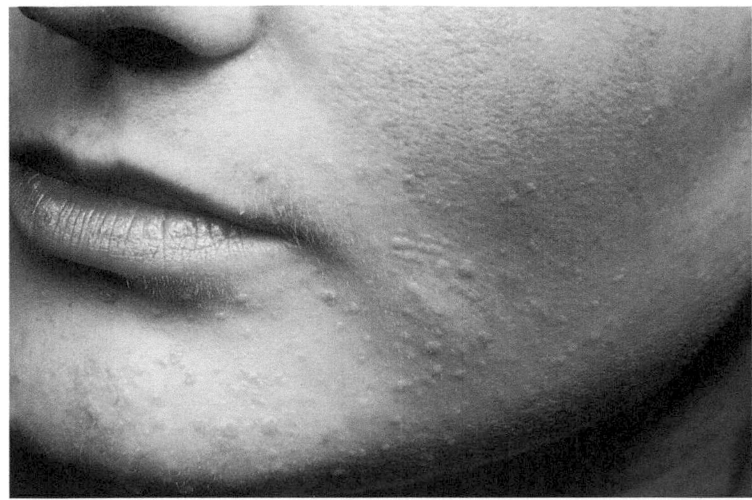

Figure 10.12

Plane warts affecting skin of lower jaw.

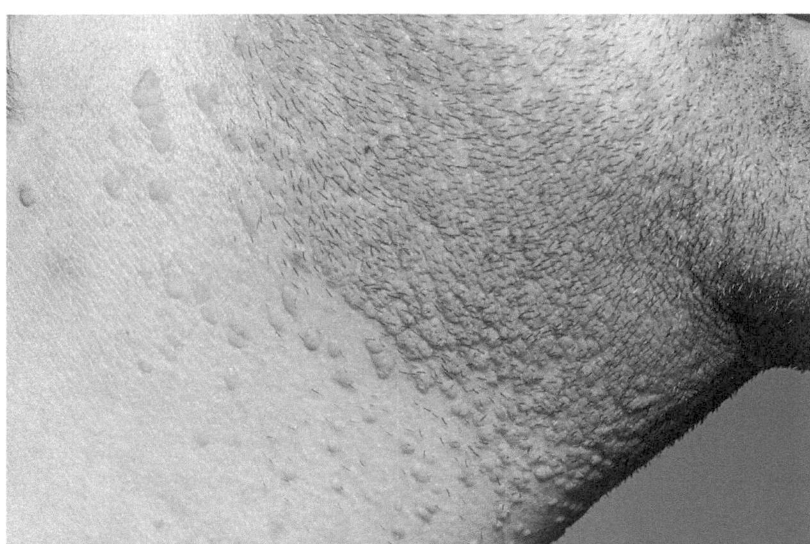

Figure 10.12a

Dense plane warts on jaw and upperneck in immunosuppressed individual.

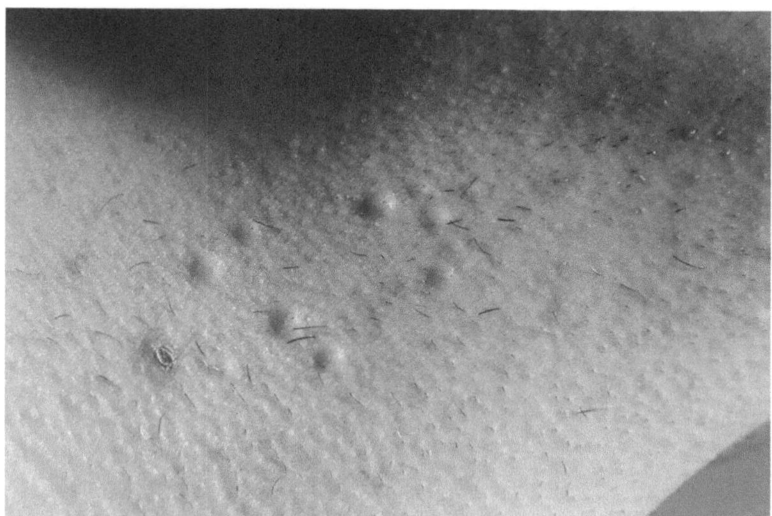

Figure 10.13

Typical molluscum contagiosum lesions.

immunodeficiency and have been reported as a particular problem of HIV-infected homosexual men.[16] MC is also more prolific in patients with atopic dermatitis and, curiously, they sometimes appear to develop eczematous areas around themselves. As with warts, they spontaneously resolve and sometimes cause considerable inflammation when they do.

Management

These lesions are best left to spontaneously resolve. If 'action' is needed, then, as with warts, if great care is used to avoid the normal skin, strong salicylic acid preparations can be employed for a few days. Topical imiquimod (5%) can also be used.

References

1. Koning S, Mohammedamin RS, van der Wouden JC. Impetigo: incidence and treatment in Dutch general practice in 1987 and 2001 – results from two national surveys. Br J Dermatol 2006; 154: 239–43.
2. Kuniyuki S, Nakano K, Maekawa N, Suzuki S. Topical antibiotic treatment of impetigo with tetracycline. J Dermatol 2005; 32: 788–92.
3. Bonnetblanc JM, Bedane. Erysipelas: recognition and management. Am J Clin Dermatol 2003; 4: 157–63.
4. Ormerod P, Campbell I. Chemotherapy and management of tuberculosis in the United Kingdom: recommendations 1998. Thorax 1998; 53: 536–48.
5. Pravda DJ, Pugliese MM. Tinea faciei. Arch Dermatol 1978; 114: 250–2.
6. Lin RL, Szepietowski JC, Schwartz RA. Tinea faciei, an often deceptive facial eruption. Int J Dermatol 2004; 43: 437–40.
7. Marks R, Dawber RPR. In situ microbiology of the stratum corneum. Arch Dermatol 1972; 105: 216–21.
8. Gorani A, Oriani A, Cambiaghi S. Seborrhoeic dermatitis like tinea faciei. Pediatr Dermatol 2005; 22: 243–4.
9. Ire AF, Marks R. Tinea incognito. Br Med J 1968; 3: 149–52.
10. Atzori L, Ferreli C, Zucca M et al. Facial cellulitis associated with Pseudomonas

aeruginosa complicating ophthalmic herpes zoster. Dermatol Online J 2004; 10: 20.

11. Darragh TM, Egbert BM, Berger TG, Yen TS. Identification of herpes simplex virus DNA in lesions of erythema pultiforme by the polymerase chain reaction. J Am Dermatol 1991; 24: 23–6.
12. Corey L, Wald A. New developments in the biology of genital herpes. In: Sacks SL, Strauss SE, Whitley RJ, Giffiths PD, eds. Clinical Management of Herpes Virus Infections. Amsterdam: TOS Press, 1995: 43–53.
13. Opstelten W, Zaal JW. Managing herpes zoster in primary care. BMJ 2005; 331: 147–51.
14. Pollock B, Highet AS. An interesting response to sensitization on facial warts. Diphencyprone (DPC) treatment for viral warts. J Dermatolog Treat 2002; 13: 47–50.
15. Hagman JH, Bianchi L, Marulli GC et al. Successful treatment of multiple filiform facial warts with imiquimod 5% cream in a patient infected by human immunodeficiency virus. Clin Exp Dermatol 2003; 28: 260–1.
16. Kolokotronis A, Antoniades D, Katsoulidis E, Kioses V. Facial and perioral molluscum contagiosum as a manifestation of HIV infection. Aust Dent J 2000; 45: 49–52.

Index

N.B. Page numbers in *italic* indicate material in figures and tables.

T - #0528 - 071024 - C188 - 246/189/9 - PB - 9780367389390 - Gloss Lamination